Dying for a Drink

7/20/12

Dr. Dier —
I hope
you enjoy
Sandy

J.

Dying for a Drink

◆

The Hidden Epidemic of Alcoholism

Dr. Santi Meunier

iUniverse, Inc.
New York Lincoln Shanghai

Dying for a Drink
The Hidden Epidemic of Alcoholism

Copyright © 2008 by Dr. Santi Meunier

iUniverse books may be ordered through booksellers or by contacting:

iUniverse
2021 Pine Lake Road, Suite 100
Lincoln, NE 68512
www.iuniverse.com
1-800-Authors (1-800-288-4677)

ISBN: 978-0-595-47396-0 (pbk)
ISBN: 978-0-595-91674-0 (ebk)

Printed in the United States of America

Every bondsman in his own hand bears the power to cancel his captivity.

William Shakespeare

Contents

Introduction

No one is immune to the negative effects of alcohol abuse. We as a global society experience the negative effects of alcohol and alcoholism socially, morally, and financially. Anne Schaef, in her book, *When Society Becomes an Addict,* calls our society 'an addictive system': a system in denial, with tunnel vision, much like that of an alcoholic.[1] What, we might ask, will it take to "wake up" to the fact that alcohol abuse is putting a tremendous strain on our nation's economy? There are over 20 million alcoholics in the United States and hundreds of thousands die each year as a result of their addiction.[2] The costs of alcoholism in the U.S. soar past $300 billion a year, and that figure is rising[3].

Alcoholics fill our prisons and hospitals. Alcohol-related crimes, fires, motor vehicle accidents, physical and mental health-related issues, lost production in the workplace and in our schools, and welfare and social programs all contribute to the rising cost, and this does not include the numbers of people suffering undiagnosed alcoholism. Alcoholism is the number two killer in this country behind cancer.[4] Many believe that the statistics are even higher, as the costs for treatment of many of the physical complications arising in middle and late stages of the disease are not often included in alcoholism-related statistics. Often, alcoholism is not cited as the "cause of death" on the death certificate. It is a startling fact that about only 14% of the deaths caused by alcoholism are so labeled. Suicide and drinking-related accidents make up about one third of deaths identified as alcohol-related.[5]

The statistics speak for themselves as to the enormity and pervasiveness of the diseases of alcoholism and addiction. According to Schaef, "The addictive system invites us to become co-dependent, to refuse to see people and things as they are. It is only when people are seen as they are that they can accept and take responsibility for themselves."[6] This rampant state of denial has infiltrated not only the alcoholic and his or her family, but the alcoholic's employer, community, and society as a whole. It is a silent and deadly epidemic that is putting a tremendous strain on the entire global community. More needs to be done to alleviate the suffering caused by this crisis. A nation united in its support for recovery from alcoholism and addiction begins with understanding the disease and our personal responsibility with it. If every individual commits to being part of the solution within his/her sphere, the tide will begin to turn on this enormous problem.

The "disease" of alcoholism is no longer thought of as a subjective diagnosis, but as a medical diagnosis of a brain disorder. Perhaps viewing a brain scan of an active alcoholic and seeing the organic differences between an alcoholic's brain and one of a normal drinker would help to demystify the disease and lift the moral judgments placed alcoholics since the beginning. Psychological, cultural, and social factors play important roles in the alcoholic's drinking behaviors and patterns, although they do not determine whether that person will become an alcoholic. The person's physiology determines whether he/she will become addicted to alcohol. Many factors contribute to this—and more are being discovered—but it has been clearly established that the alcoholic's genetic make-up, hormones, brain chemistry and enzymes all play a role in the development of the disease. It is important for psychotherapists and physicians in the field of addiction to be open to new forms of treatment based on the latest scientific discoveries if we are to reach a larger number of sick and suffering alcoholics and effectively help them.

Alcoholism is not curable but it is treatable. Alcoholics who abstain from drinking alcohol may halt the physical part of the disease. The mental, emotional, behavioral and spiritual features of the disease are more complex, to treat, but millions of sober alcoholics all over the world speak to the efficacy of Alcoholics Anonymous as well as that of other holistic treatment models. At present, significant scientific technology and research is focused on exploring ancient techniques and practices to better understand the sources of their healing potential and how they may used to treat diseases such as alcoholism. Candace Pert, a research professor and author of the best selling book, *Molecules of Emotion*, explains, "Hypnosis, yogic breathing, and many energy-based therapies (ranging from bioenergetics and other psychotherapies centered on body work to chiropractic, massage and therapeutic touch) provide examples of techniques that can be used to effect change at a level beneath consciousness." [7]

Elmer Green, the Mayo Clinic physician and a pioneer in the use of biofeedback for treating an array of diseases writes, "Every change in the physiological state is accompanied by an appropriate change in the mental emotional state, conscious or unconscious, and conversely, every change in the mental emotional state, conscious or unconscious, is accompanied by an appropriate change in the physiological state." [8] The latest research into the role of neuropeptides (chemical substances made primarily by brain cells) and the body's chemistry of emotion may prove to be an important key to understanding the role our thoughts and feelings play in the healing of many diseases. Equally important is the scientific exploration and discovery of the true efficacy of many ancient healing modalities and how they may affect the development of future medical treatments.

Dr. Joseph Volpicelli and the U.S. Substance Abuse and Mental Health Services Administration states, "20 million Americans suffer from alcohol abuse disorders, yet only about 2 million are in any kind of treatment program. We should be flexible enough to get at the 90% who are not in treatment." [9]

I feel strongly that the current trend of scientific research will prove to have a tremendous effect on the identification, treatment, and stabilization of the disease of alcoholism in the next decade. I plan to continue my research into the cause and effects of alcoholism on the individual, the family, and the country. I am very hopeful that the tide is turning on this epidemic and that we may all one day see a primarily sober society where alcoholism is diagnosed and treated at the level that it exists, and that no alcoholic falls through the cracks of denial again.

1

THE LURE OF ALCOHOL

Alcohol is a product of amazing versatility.
It will remove stains from designer clothes.
It will also remove the clothes off your back.
If it is used in sufficient quantity, Alcohol will
Remove the furniture from your home, also
Rugs from the floor, food from the table,
Lining from the stomach, vision from the eyes,
And judgment from the mind.
Alcohol will remove good reputations,
Good jobs, good friends, happiness from children's hearts.
Sanity, freedom, spouses, relationships,
One's ability to adjust and live with fellow man,
And even life itself.
As a remover of things, alcohol has no equal.

Anonymous

Alcohol is as old as time itself, and yet it still remains a mysterious substance. It is the only drug that can be classified as a food, though one rich in calories and energizing effects, but deficient in vitamins and minerals. When used in small amounts it produces a stimulating effect; when ingested in larger amounts it acts as a sedative. Surprisingly, perhaps, alcohol is not considered an addiction-producing drug by the World Health Organization (WHO). An addiction-producing drug, according to researchers James Milam and Katherine Ketcham, is one that creates an irresistible need in most users, an increased tolerance for the drug, and mild to painful withdrawal symptoms.[10] To any alcoholic, alcohol would seem to fit these criteria. In point of fact, Milam and Ketcham found that alcohol

1

is addictive to only about 10% of its users, compared to heroin, which is addictive to 100% of its users.[11] Alcohol, it may therefore be argued, belongs in a category by itself.

Alcohol the Potentially Addictive Drug

Alcohol has addictive as well as habit-forming properties, and millions of people become psychologically and emotionally dependent on it. The two researchers cite that over 100 million people drink alcohol in the United States and approximately 10 million of them are alcoholics.[12] When used by alcoholics, alcohol meets the criteria for classification as an addiction-producing drug.

The alcoholic drinks in the beginning to feel good, but as the addiction progresses he or she will drink to escape the painful withdrawal of not drinking. The craving is so strong and relentless that a malnourished alcoholic will crave alcohol over food. This creates a downward spiral that can eventually lead to death. Understanding alcohol, the drug, is crucial to understanding its potentially lethal effect on the physical body.

Ethyl alcohol or ethanol has been called "the excrement of yeast", as it is understood to consume sweets (glucose) and subsequently release an enzyme that converts the sugars into carbon dioxide (CO_2) and alcohol (CH_3CH_2OH) in a process known as fermentation. The yeast "feeds" voraciously on the sugars until it has acute alcohol "intoxication", at which point it dies.[13] How ironic that yeast and alcoholics experience the same fate. Louis Pasteur discovered that fermentation is the fungi's act of survival. The yeast needs the grain—for example, barley malt—in order to release enzymes that convert starches into simple sugars.

Distillation was discovered in Arabia around A.D.800. The word alcohol comes from the Arabic word "alkuhl" which means essence.[14] It is probable that humans discovered ethanol in prehistoric times in the form of fermented fruit juices which then became wines, or malted grains which were used in making beer. Ethanol is most likely as old as life itself. Perhaps the problem of over-consumption is as well. Even as early as the 16th century the anatomical studies conducted by Vesalius recognized that an abuse of alcoholic beverages was associated with diseases such as those affecting the liver. Ironically, it has been only recently that certain liver diseases have a clear link to alcohol abuse and not to the malnutrition associated with heavy drinking, as it had been in the past. The debate as to whether alcohol is toxic to the human body has been intense and long-lived, not just among the general public but also among physicians and professionals. As recently as 1949, renowned physiologist Charles Best wrote, "there is no more evidence of a specific toxic effect of pure ethyl alcohol upon liver than there is due to sugar". The debate surrounding the deadly effects of alcohol consumption therefore continues—five hundred years after Vesalius's findings.

It has been only in recent memory that the deadly effects of cigarette smoking have been exposed. Peer pressure has demoted cigarette smoking from glamorous and "cool" to gauche and distasteful. Smokers now have to get their "fix" in the back alleys of fine restaurants where smoking is no longer permitted inside. Cigarette smoking has thus declined since it peaked in 1981 when Americans smoked 640 billion cigarettes. The lethal effects of alcohol are just as preventable as those of smoking. It is perhaps a statement more about our addictive nature as human beings that we are reluctant to "give up" substances that give us pleasure—regardless of the consequences. The scientific facts abound regarding these addictive substances; what is lacking is perhaps the willingness to accept those facts as reality.

The use of the term "proof" with alcoholic beverages began in 17th century England through the practice of proving strength in a drink by mixing it with gunpowder and seeing if it would ignite. A drink containing 49% alcohol could be ignited. This means that a whiskey that is 86 proof is 43% alcohol, that is, alcohol comprises approximately 49–50% of its total volume of contents.[15]

In its pure state, ethanol alcohol is colorless, but delivers a burning, unpalatable taste. It must be combined with various substances called 'congeners' to make it more appealing for consumption. Congeners give us the variety of types of alcoholic beverages, but they also give us additives about which we consumers may be unaware. Congeners contain trace amounts of inorganic substances such as aluminum, silicon and lead, to name only a few. Milam & Ketcham point out that alcoholic beverages often also contain methyl, fusel oil, lactic acids, ketones, propyl, carbon dioxide and more.[16] Heavy drinkers may, therefore, unknowingly consume unhealthy amounts of these substances, several of which are actually poisonous in higher quantities.

What Happens When A Person Drinks?

When a person has a drink of alcohol, it first irritates the tissue in the mouth and esophagus before passing to the stomach, where approximately 20% of the alcohol enters the bloodstream and is carried throughout the body. Within minutes, the alcohol reaches the brain, slowing down and numbing its function. Long-term heavy drinking actually causes brain degeneration and produces signs of atrophy. Alcohol is metabolized mostly in the liver, where enzymes convert ethanol, the toxifying agent in alcohol, into carbon dioxide and water. It takes the liver one hour to metabolize one-third of an ounce of alcohol. Nothing will alter this process in the liver, contrary to the myth that a pot of hot coffee will counteract the metabolism of alcohol and sober up the drunk. Heavy alcohol consumption causes the liver to become fatty and enlarged over time, and can lead to cirrhosis, a chronic disease of the liver characterized by the replacement of normal tissue with fibrous tissue. This condition can lead to liver failure and death because normal blood flow is impeded. If consumption continues, speech, balance, vision and decision-making become impaired. Chronic consumption can lead to what is commonly known as a "black-out" where the user does not remember a period of time even though she may appear to be alert to others. If drinking continues, it can lead to the loss of consciousness. Socrates observed centuries ago, "If we pour ourselves immense droughts, it will be no long time before our bodies and minds reel." When extremely high levels are ingested, alcoholic poisoning and/or respiratory failure can occur.

Alcoholism increases the risk of heart disease and various cancers. The heart pumps 35 million times per year. The heart of an alcoholic is likely to be flabby and enlarged, impairing it. Blood then accumulates in the lungs, causing edema, or excess fluid. The heart can become so riddled with scar tissue that oxygen cannot be pumped through it effectively. Eventually the alcoholic may suffer a potentially fatal heart attack

The concentration of alcohol in the body is determined by the blood alcohol level (BAL). BAL is the measure of the percentage of alcohol in the blood. A reading of .05 BAL is 5 parts alcohol to 100 parts blood. A driver is legally under the influence when his/her BAL is above .08. If the driver is given a breathalyzer test and registers .08 -.10 he/she is charged with drunk driving.[17] The BAL is affected by weight, sex, and age so these variables are considered when assessing an individual case.

Alcohol is a depressant to the central nervous system. It depresses both the inhibitory and excitatory neurons. This is why some people will experience an excitable high from drinking, while others may become very maudlin and lethargic. Intoxication comes from the altering of neuronal transmissions across nerve cells. This is why when an alcoholic takes a drink he will likely feel quickly relieved of distressful withdrawal-related symptoms, including tremors, which the alcohol will reduce or stop altogether. This altering of neural activity increases the sense of pleasure, but actually negatively impacts physical capacity. William Shakespeare, a keen observer of human emotions and behavior, once wrote, "It provokes the desire, but it takes away the performance".

The Phenomenon of Addiction

What is addiction and who is at risk? Why do some people seem predisposed to addiction, while others appear to be immune to the effects of pleasurable substances? Studies in brain research and the biochemistry of addiction are building a deeper understanding of the destructive addiction process. Addiction to pleasure-producing chemicals is not new. As Margaret Hamburg pointed out in her 1986 Vogue Magazine article, *The Nature of Craving,* the Sumerians used opium six thousand years ago, and created a written symbol for it meaning "joy".[18] Anthropologists trained Rhesus monkeys in a lab to press a lever for a reward. The monkeys demonstrated that they were willing to press the lever four thousand times for a single dose of cocaine. In other experiments, rats and monkeys chose cocaine over food and nourishment.

According to Dr. Hamburg, these important experiments led scientists to suspect a mechanism for addiction within our brain. She describes the studies of James Olds, who observed how the insertion of electrodes deep into specific areas of an animal's brain triggered the animal's drive to repeat the electronic stimulation continuously for hours.[19]

Behaviors that result in pleasure or reward are referred to as positive reinforcement. This function is normal and vital in reinforcing key pleasurable behaviors essential to sustained life such as eating, drinking, and propagation. Alcohol and other drugs of abuse (AOD's) can act as chemical surrogates that induce a euphoric state the mind will wish to repeat.[20] These drugs may become more powerfully rewarding than the natural positive reinforcements like eating or sleeping, as the brain seeks to recreate that pleasurable mental state. Addiction occurs when the person seeks the AOD's before and eventually instead of the natural ones. Once alcohol-seeking behavior is established, the brain will adapt in order to continue functioning despite the disruptive effects of the alcohol. As alcohol consumption continues, the individual can then become dependent on the substance in order to avoid feelings of discomfort and/or cravings. Now the brain has switched from seeking to re-create pleasure from the drug to avoiding the painful stimuli of withdrawal. Negative and positive reinforcements are now in effect for the alcoholic.[21]

A person is physically dependent on alcohol when the need for consumption is driven by a withdrawal syndrome. This generally occurs 6–48 hours after the last drink. The withdrawal syndrome is the result of the adaptation of the nervous system to the effects of alcohol. Symptoms can include anxiety, anger, agitation, tremor, elevated blood pressure and, in the most extreme cases, seizures.[22]

Ironically, many of the emotional withdrawal symptoms that occur from alcohol abuse are the very same feelings that many people experienced prior to alcohol dependence. Alcohol acts to relieve the stress that it created in the first place. The same feelings of isolation, anxiety, boredom, depression, trauma, crisis, or self-centered fears such as low self esteem, abandonment and inadequacy are now the trigger mechanisms for continued alcohol abuse. This vicious cycle frequently spirals downward, producing deeper and deeper feelings of despair.

Dr. Archibald Hart in his 1990 book, "Healing Life's Hidden Addictions" speaks of the two major drives that underlie the addictive process: seeking to increase excitement and reduce tension. Trigger mechanisms are the stimuli that set off these two drives. The addict will seek to "medicate" these feelings using the AOD's upon which the brain has become dependent. Dr. Hart says that the major trigger for many addicts stems from selfish needs commonly called "polarized narcissism". He believes that this state is often found in people who have suffered from early trauma where their dependency needs were not properly met, leading to a drive for instant gratification. Addictive personalities want what they want when they want it. Anything that threatens failure, abandonment, rejection, or fear can trigger the addictive cycle.

Denial plays a very important role in the fostering of addiction. The addict is often the last to realize that he/she has a problem. Alcoholics Anonymous states that it is a disease that tells the alcoholic that she does not have it. The brain is so invested in reinforcing the need for the addictive chemical to counteract the pain of withdrawal that the subconscious mind blocks awareness of the dependency from the conscious mind. Denial is a kind of survival mechanism for the mind while being a dangerous tool for the progression of the addiction. Dr. Hart believes that the more unconscious the connection between the need and the behavior that brings about the relief, the more powerful the addiction. Denial must be lifted and the addict fully aware of his/her malady if abstinence is to be possible. The first step in Alcoholics Anonymous speaks to just this issue, "We realized that we were powerless over alcohol and that our lives had become unmanageable". Awareness of the addiction, which seems so obvious to the observer, can elude many an addict right into the grave. Anyone who loves or knows someone who is addicted must understand that because of the strong denial component, attempts to reach an addict through logic is completely ineffective. You will never permeate the defenses. Only the addict, from an inner awareness of the truth, can break down the denial inherent in the addiction.

Alcohol and the Brain

All brain function involves communication among the neurons in the brain. Each neuron communicates with other neurons and through the movement of chemicals called neurotransmitters across synaptic spaces between each neuron. There are approximately 100 neurotransmitters in the human brain. Scientists are currently attempting to identify the communication processes of neurotransmitters and subtype receptors in the addict's brain as a first step in developing effective medications for alcoholism treatment.[23]

Dr. Nora Volkow, the director of the National Institute on Drug Abuse (NIDA), believes that addiction may be a malfunction of the normal human craving for stimulation, vitality and the powerful feeling of being fully alive. This understanding has led researchers to identify and investigate the brain chemical, dopamine. Dopamine is a neurochemical long understood to be involved in motivation, pleasure, and learning. It is commonly referred to as the body's "reward button". Research has shown that addictive substances like cocaine and nicotine increase the production of dopamine in the brain. It was therefore assumed that, with the increase of dopamine in the brain as a result of ingesting addictive drugs, addicts should be in a perpetual state of euphoria. This holds true in the early stages of addiction, and many an alcoholic will go on for years chasing the memory of that early blissful experience.

This is obviously not the case as alcoholism and drug addiction progress with worsening effects particularly in view of the high rate of chronic depression among addicts. It is currently believed that approximately one third of alcoholic deaths are from suicides or accidents. This is a startling number indeed. What happens in the brain of an addicted person, that despite the surge produced by the neurochemicals, the final outcome is so frequently despair and pain rather than pleasure?

In her research with the National Institute on Drug Abuse (NIDA), Director Nora D. Volkow and her team have brought new insights to the controversial theory about dopamine. In a 2004 interview with Kathleen McGowan in Psychology Today, Volkow described what she calls the salience theory of dopamine, which focuses on the neurotransmitter's function as a "survival" chemical alerting us to important information and stimuli we need to attend to in order to survive.[24] Previously the key role of dopamine was thought to be pleasure-producing. Volkow and her team noted that in addicts, dopamine levels surge 5 to 10 times more forcefully through the nucleus accumbens, the reward structure of the brain, forcing full attention on the drug—alcohol in this case—that triggered this response. Alcohol then becomes a salient need, that is, strikingly conspicuous for survival, and for the addict, it edges out other needs for food, sex, work, safety, health and, ultimately, life itself. Volkow's research has also shown in brain imagery that addicts have fewer D2 receptors, which results in a desensitizing of the dopamine system. This could explain why addicts need more and more drugs to feel anything at all. In addition to the fewer D2 receptors, brain imaging reveals that the prefrontal cortex also stops functioning normally. The prefrontal cortex is the part of the brain associated with inhibitions, judgment and control.[25] Is it possible that one thing that separates a normal drinker from an alcoholic is that the alcoholic has a sluggish dopamine circuitry and that the alcohol serves as a jump start on the system? In an alcoholic, the neurons start pumping once alcohol is taken into the body and a false sense of well-being is then experienced, however short in duration it may be.

Scientists are now realizing that pleasure seeking is just one part of the dopamine receptor system. For example when Ritalin is given to people with Attention Deficit Disorder (ADD) they are more able to concentrate. Ritalin boosts dopamine production and therefore makes it easier for the individual to focus on any given situation because in point of fact, the task becomes more interesting. Gregory Berns, Associate Professor of Psychiatry and Behavioral Science at Emory University in Atlanta suggested in the *Psychology Today* article on Volkow[26] that "Neurons really exist to process information. That's what neurons do. If you want to anthropomorphize neurons, you can say that they are happiest when they are processing information."[27] In light of this research it could be postulated that, to an alcoholic, the information transmitted by the neuron is that alcohol is the best thing in the world and it should be used above all else. Ann Arbor psychology professor Terry Robinson sums up the addictive cycle when he states, "You have enhanced motivation for the drug, and you have impaired prefrontal cortical systems. So you want the drug pathologically, and you have reduced control of behavior, and what you've got is an addict."[28]

A Natural High

In the last two decades researchers have devoted a great deal of study to endorphins, naturally-occurring, opiate-like substances in the body. When the body experiences extreme situations of stress and/or pain, it creates more endorphins to compensate for the discomfort. The endorphins act in much the same way as heroine and morphine, and so are considered the body's natural opiate system.

Researchers believe that the runner's "high" is the result of over production of endorphins by the body to compensate for the stress of strenuous exercise. Some runners have been known to become addicted to running and even experience a depression or irritability when they are not able to run. This is thought to be the result of lowered levels of endorphin production in the body.

In an addict endorphin production becomes compromised. Naturally the endorphins occupy many of the body's opiate receptors. If narcotics are taken repeatedly the body begins to reduce endorphin production in order to compensate for the opiate supply that is being ingested. Over time the brain's receptors become dependent on the outside supply of opiates and if it is not satisfied a craving will occur. This is a predominate symptom in opiate withdrawal and it can become quite severe.

Dr. Margaret Hamburg, who, has done extensive neurochemical research on addiction, believes that addiction is not a moral problem but rather a problem that stems from the brain's pleasure and pain centers. In her studies she has found that withdrawal from narcotics is accompanied by an increased activity in the nerve centers of the brain called the locus coeruleus (LC). It is in the LC that the addict experiences withdrawal symptoms. Researchers have discovered that Clonidine, a drug used to treat hypertension, has been found to lower the LC activity in opiate-addicted lab rats. Clonidine also helps some addicts ease the withdrawal symptoms of narcotics, cigarette and alcohol withdrawal as well. It is hoped that further research into brain responses to opiates, will lead to the development of more effective medications for alleviating withdrawal and enabling abstinence.

Alcohol, the Problem

Alcohol is the most widely used drug in the world and is by far the most devastating. Alcohol ruins families, friendships, jobs, health and the individual's self-esteem. It fills jails at an alarming rate. According to the National Institute on Alcohol Abuse 50% of violent crimes, 57% of incidents of spousal abuse by men, 60% of sexual offenses, and 86% of convicted murderers were found to have been drinking when they committed the crimes. It has been proposed that a beer tax of just 10% could act as a deterrent, possibly serving to help reduce the rate of murder, rape, and robbery.[29] In the 1990's, America spent approximately 136 billion dollars on alcohol-related health costs, labor issues, and crimes. Nearly 100,000 Americans die each year as a result of alcohol abuse. Motor vehicle accidents claim approximately 65,000 lives annually, of which roughly 22,000 have been identified as drunken driving accidents.[30] Sweden's tough drunk driving laws (driving with a BAC of .2 is illegal) have dramatically reduced drunken driving deaths, although they have not reduced the rate of alcoholism. Tough legislation on dangerous alcoholic behavior is very important to more effectively protect the population, but it does not address the issue of the individual alcoholic and what is required for treatment of his or her disease.

According to the 2001–2002 National Epidemiologic Survey on Alcohol and Related Conditions (NESARC), directed by the National Institute on Alcohol Abuse and Alcoholism (NIAAA), the number of American adults who abuse alcohol rose from 13.8 million to 17.6 million since 1991–1992. The NESARC study showed that while the rate of alcohol abuse increased from 3.03 to 4.65%, the rate of alcoholism decreased from 4.38 to 3.81%. The study also shows that alcohol abuse and alcoholism are now higher among white men than Hispanics, Blacks, Asians and women in general, although increases over the years prior to the study were particularly pronounced among Black and Hispanic men and Asian women ages 18–29. Dr. Bridgett Grant, who led the NESARC research team, observed, "That alcohol abuse seems to be increasing presents intriguing, clear evidence that no single societal or environmental cause can explain the increase. Further research is an important priority." [31] The full NESARC study appears in the June, 2004 issue of Drug and Alcohol Dependence (Volume 74, Number 3, pages 223–234.

2

THE GLOBAL REACH OF ALCOHOLISM

Ethnic Susceptibilities

Alcohol abuse affects all age groups, males and females, all socio-economic levels, and, religions and cultures. No one is immune from developing an addiction, but some ethnic groups have better odds of avoiding addiction than others might. Genetic researchers have discovered, for example, that approximately half of Asians carry an altered gene that impairs their ability to process alcohol, which causes unpleasant physical effects. In his exhaustive 1992 National Geographic report, *The Legal Addiction*, Gibbons describes what happens when the enzyme that normally metabolizes acetaldehyde becomes inactive at the site of the genetic alteration: an increase in the toxic acetaldehyde ensues, leading the user to experience sweating, flushing and nausea that can be very severe.[32] (It is ironic, however, that even in light of this strong deterrent, social pressures caused a virtual explosion in problem drinking in Asia.) Gibbon's noted that the Japanese consumed twice as much alcohol in the late eighties and early nineties as they had in the 1950's. On the other hand, among Italians, Gibbons estimated that only 9% of the population in Italy was alcoholic and the numbers had been declining during the years preceding his 1992 article. This held true at the time as well for the French even though they were the heaviest drinkers among the groups surveyed. The Hungarians, however, had doubled their drinking since the 1970's, with deaths from cirrhosis increasing five-fold in the prior 30 years.[33] The Gibbons study noted that Russians have been in the grip of alcoholism throughout their history. Grand Prince Vladimir had once touted that "drinking is the joy of Russia", while incidents of alcoholic poisoning continued to rise until 1985 when Mikhail Gorbachev enforced a prohibition of sorts to try to stabilize the nation's alcoholic death rate of 40,000 per year.[34]

At the time of their research, Milam & Ketcham reported that the Jews had a very low rate of alcoholism at 1%, even though as a culture they have been exposed to alcohol for over 7,000 years.[35] Native Americans, on the other hand, suffered the highest statistics for alcoholism and related problems, including fetal alcoholic syndrome, traumatic deaths and cirrhosis. In 1992 they were rated as 3 times the national average.[36] This is a staggering rate of 80–90%.[37]

Alcohol in America

An Historical Perspective

America is the "melting pot" of many cultures, customs, and religions and therefore reflects a dynamic configuration of attitudes regarding alcohol and alcohol abuse. Many of the beliefs and prejudices about drinking and problem drinkers have prevailed since the early eighteenth and nineteenth centuries. Despite scientific research revealing the physical and mental disease of alcoholism, society as a whole still views alcohol and drug abuse as a moral issue and a sign of weakness and instability. In order to fully understand this deeply ingrained attitude it is important to review the history of alcohol use in America.[38]

The colonists from England practiced long-established rituals regarding alcohol, using it for religious, medicinal, and nutritional purposes. Until the 1700's, alcohol production and consumption, then generally in the form of beer and wine, was centered in the family system. As the distilling industry grew and the distribution of distilled spirits expanded throughout the country, alcohol production and use went from being a family centered activity to primarily a male social activity. In the Colonies, the majority of problem drinkers were young men, and as a result, intoxicated destructive behavior became a major social concern. By the end of the eighteenth century 90% of the alcohol that was consumed was in the form of distilled spirits and in 1807 it was recorded that in Boston alone there was a distillery for every 40 inhabitants. The increasing demand for alcohol and the abusive behaviors that followed it moved sober citizens to establish the temperance movement, which grew in popularity, peaking in the 1830's with over a million active members.[39]

Alcohol: The Crisis

危
机
The Chinese symbol for crisis is made up of two characters: danger and opportunity. Concerns and judgments regarding the problem drinker and the effects on society are as old as our nation, but the threat is reaching epidemic proportions. The need to arm ourselves with medical, psychological, and social information is paramount if we are to truly understand the issues surrounding addiction. Easy access to inexpensive narcotics and peer pressure has led to a younger and younger addicted population. It is a crisis, and we as a nation need to embrace the reality of this crisis in order to overcome it.

I believe that, as a nation, how we choose to deal with this crisis will bear a tremendous effect on the future. Our young people are at risk, and they need for us to act wisely and firmly in finding solutions to this destructive problem. We will either deal with our nation's addiction problem or the addiction problem will deal with us.

Alcohol Use and Abuse

"Why are you drinking?" demanded the little prince.
"So that I may forget," replied the tippler.
"Forget what?" inquired the little prince, who already was sorry for him.
"Forget that I am ashamed," the tippler confessed, hanging his head.
"Ashamed of what?" insisted the little prince, who wanted to help him.
"Ashamed of my drinking!" The tippler brought his speech to an end, and shut himself up in an impregnable silence.

Antoine de Saint-Exup`ery, The Little Prince

Alcohol and alcoholism have invaded every aspect of our society. Abusers are getting younger and younger. Addiction is present in every socio-economic class and culture, ethnicity and religion. Alcoholism is thought to be by many professionals the number one killer in America and yet the funds for research and treatment are low in proportion to the problem. So the problems of alcohol abuse and addiction continue to increase, and the acts of denial and/or moral judgments about whether or not alcoholism is really a disease persist. It seems that no one can escape the effects of alcohol abuse and alcoholism. Ask anyone if he or she has now, or has ever had a loved one, colleague, or family member who suffers the ravages of chronic alcohol abuse. This is a national crisis, and we can see it as an opportunity to look deeply at the cultural quagmire and begin to address the serious and dangerous issues that lurk within it.

Drinking Games

Beer ping pong is a popular game among college students. The game promises a "buzz" to end all buzzes. Ping pong balls are flung into tumblers filled with beer, and the loser has to chug-a-lug the tumblers. The amount of alcohol that can be consumed in a short period of time is in lethal proportions. Student drinking games are a part of college life, and far too often, a deadly part of it. MIT student Scott Krueger drank himself to death in 1997. The celebrations around sports have also been a tragic arena for lethal drinking. The Red Sox extraordinary win of the World Series in 2004 was no exception.

Since 1993, the percentage of binge-drinking among college students has remained at an alarming 44%. It is likely to become much higher.[40] College students die from drinking at an alarming rate as well. In 2004, 1,400 campus deaths were attributed to alcohol abuse. Colleges across the nation are instituting recovery dorms for students who want a sober environment or are in a treatment group such as Alcoholics Anonymous.

Alcohol abusers are getting younger and younger

According to the 1998 National Household Survey on Drug Abuse (NHSDA), sponsored by the Substance Abuse & Mental Health Service Administration (SAMHSA), 19% of the boys between 12 and 17 have used alcohol in the past month. Nearly 3 in 10 (29%) consume six or more alcoholic beverages each time they drink. The average age of a boy's first drink of alcohol is 11 years. Teenage boys who drink take more risks with girls, engage in binge drinking, use marijuana together with alcohol and are more likely to drink and drive.

Risk Factors for Boys Who Use Alcohol [1]

- Boys may be more susceptible to a family history of alcoholism than girls are. (McGue, 1991, p. 22#)

---

1. The following online reports provide additional information and sources on risk factors for boys who use alcohol: for example: www.simmons.edu/ssw/sls/alcohol_dependence.ppt

- Boys develop attention deficit disorder (ADD) and Attention Deficit Hyperactivity Disorder (ADHD) at a higher rate than girls. ADHD can be a strong predictor of early-onset drinking problems.

- Thirty percent of high school aged boys who were sexually or physically abused reported they were drinking, sometimes heavily (5 or more drinks in a row on at least 5 days in a month period). Boys who had not reported being abused but who drank heavily was only at 16%.

- High school-aged boys engage in riskier sexual practices, and 39% say it is acceptable to force girls who are drunk to have sex.

- Among heavy teenage drinkers boys were more likely than girls to say that they drink because they do not believe they will live long enough to face the risks.

- Teenage boys are more likely to drive after binge drinking than are girls or older boys.

Alcohol Abuse by Girls

Girls are beginning to drink at younger and younger ages as well. According to SAMHSA"s 1998 survey 38% of girl's ages 12 through 17 reported using alcohol. The risk factors for girls are somewhat different than for boys. One study found symptoms of depression among teenage drinking girls 50% higher than in teenage boys. Among 8th grade girls who drink heavily, 37% reported attempting suicide compared to 11% who said they do not drink.

Risk Factors for Girls Who Use Alcohol [2]

- Girls are at greater risk of depression during puberty than boys. One in four girls who drank had symptoms of depression.

- Girls are more likely to succumb to peer pressure, often being introduced to alcohol by older boy friends.

- Girls are more likely than boys to drink to escape problems and frustrations.

- Girls who have been sexually abused are 50% more likely to abuse alcohol.

---

2. For more information on alcohol use and associated risk factors among girls, visit www.health.org/govpubs/rpo993

- Sustained heavy drinking has been associated with menstrual problems, some leading to infertility.

- Two-thirds of rapes and sexual assaults among young people involve alcohol.

The statistics are troubling, and provide indications of ways family predisposition can increase the likelihood of teenage drinking. Both sons and daughters of alcoholics are at a greater risk of problem drinking during adolescence and of possibly developing alcoholism later in life. The media also plays a role. Although large tobacco and alcohol companies deny targeting young people, the elements of certain print ads and commercials clearly appeal to the youth market. The Beer Institute donates money to 75 substance abuse programs, and four out of every five safe drinking messages on television are funded by beer companies.[41] Their apparent intention is to warn young people against using alcohol, but the statistics speak louder than words. Girls are beginning to drink at younger and younger ages and the numbers of girls who begin drinking between the ages of 10–14 have risen 31% in the last thirty years.[42] The average age for boys who first try alcohol is age eleven.[43] The bottom line is, would the beer and cigarette industry spend billions of advertising dollars annually to drive potential customers away?

An Ounce of Prevention

The Social Norms Resource Center defines a binge drinker as one who consumes more than 4 or 5 drinks in one sitting over a two-week period. In children ages 12–17 SAMSHA's (www.samsha.gov.) criteria for a heavy binge drinker would be one consuming five or more drinks in a row at least five days a month. The problem with teenage drinking is so severe that over 2,000 high schools in the country have installed intoximeters to check teens at risk for drinking problems.

Some of the behavioral symptoms for both adolescents and adults are the same. The following list is a guide of indications that a child may be using alcohol. It is important to point out that if you observe some of these symptoms it does not necessarily mean that he or she is using drugs or alcohol. Certainly further investigation should be done.

Behavioral Symptoms

- Mood swings; personality changes; defensiveness; overly emotional, self-centered; manipulative behaviors
- Strained and difficult communications
- Withdrawal from family
- Changes in dress, friends, likes and dislikes
- Lack of self-discipline; apathy; school/work problems
- Anxious behavior; fearful
- Fitful sleep patterns
- Poor coping skills; depression; anxiety
- significant change(s) in appearance, attitude, personality, or routine.

Physical Symptoms

- Fatigue; weight gain or loss
- Bloodshot watery eyes and/or dilated pupils
- Rundown condition resulting in frequent colds, sore throats, flu-like symptoms
- Nausea and/or vomiting
- Shaky hands, sweating
- Poor coordination-stumbling or dizzy spells
- Irregular heartbeat, high blood pressure
- Troubling sleeping, restless and irritable
- Temper tantrums or outburst
- Chronically inflamed nostrils, runny nose
- Always dressed in long sleeves, even in hot weather

More details on signs and symptoms can be found on the Watershed Treatment Center website at: www.thewatershed.com/signs.htm.

If you notice any of these changes, please don't put off confronting the child to find out more about what he or she is experiencing. The adolescent years are often difficult for everyone in the family. Children change and grow rapidly, and with their hormonal levels and other "growing pains" increasing, moods can take on dramatic proportions. Some of this is perfectly normal no matter how hard it is to deal with at the time. Separating what is normal from what is a danger signal is the responsibility of each parent and care-giver. There is too much to lose from ignoring the challenges. A wonderful book for any parent dealing with a difficult youngster is *TOUGHLOVE*, by Phyllis York and Ted Wachtel. The authors are both helping professionals who faced the nightmare of an out-of-control teen-aged child. They are the founders of the ToughLove movement and their book outlines what parents can do to truly help their addicted, troubled children, including advice on setting-up a parent support group.

Another educational resource that parents can use to help children avoid alcohol addiction problems is Girl Power, sponsored by the U.S. Department of Health and Human Services and developed by SAMHSA"s center for Substance Abuse Prevention. Girl Power is designed to help girls ages 9–14 to make healthier choices for themselves, and involves parents, communities, and professionals to provide education and support. Girl Power can be found on the web at: www.health.org/gpower

3

WHAT IS ALCOHOLISM?

Yesterday this day's madness did prepare;
To-morrow's silence, triumph, or despair:
Drink!—for you know not whence you came, nor why:
Drink!—for you know not why you go, nor where.

—Omar Khayyam

People have been drinking to ward off a cold, to celebrate a wedding, to cook a meal or to enhance a festivity since the Egyptians and Babylonians first crushed grapes thousands of years ago. Consumed in moderation it is a relaxing beverage with some health benefits. It is a widely used and acceptable beverage worldwide. Of the more than 100 million people in United States who drink alcohol, however, Milam & Ketcham warn in their book *Under the Influence*, "one in ten is an alcoholic."[44]

Alcoholism is ranked the number two killer in this country after cancer. However, since alcoholism is often undiagnosed as the cause of death, many experts believe that alcoholism is actually the number one killer of Americans. Milam & Ketcham estimate that currently only 14% of the deaths caused by alcoholism are diagnosed as such.[45] That means that 86% of alcoholics die before they are properly diagnosed. Many of the diseases that develop in the third and final stage of alcoholism are often what are cited as the cause of death. According to W. Schmidt and R.E. Popham's 1978 study on the causes of death in alcoholics, 24% are due to cirrhosis, 30% to cardiovascular disease, 15% to upper G.I. problems and lung cancer, 7% to pneumonia, 14% alcoholism and 10% other causes.[46] Alcoholism increases the risk of heart disease and cancer as well as liver failure.[47] Alcoholism can lead to cancer of the larynx, esophagus, stomach, pancreas, and upper gastrointestinal tract. It can damage a fetus, and, in the most extreme cases, lead to Fetal Alcohol Syndrome (FAS). The harm alcohol addiction does to the body has been known throughout the ages.

Milam & Ketcham explore historical observations about the consequences of alcoholism, and quote 19th British minister Benjamin Parsons' 1840 essay portraying alcohol as a predator to the human body:

> Among all sources of disease, alcohol stands preeminent as a destroyer ... This pestilent principal generally seeks asylum where it may practice its deadliest deeds in some important and vital organ of the body. It sometimes makes the brain the seat of its venom, and victim of its cruelties. At another time, it hides itself in the inmost recess of the heart, or coils around like a serpent; now it fixes upon the lungs; now upon the kidneys, upon the liver, the bladder, the pancreas, the intestines or the skin. It can agitate the heart until it throbs and bursts, or it can reduce pulsation until it becomes impalpable. It can distract the head until the brain sweats blood and horrified reason flies away and leaves the man a maniac or a madman ... I never knew a person become insane who was not in the habit of taking a portion of alcohol daily.[48]

When does Alcohol Abuse Become Alcoholism?

What distinguishes heavy drinkers or social drinkers from alcoholics? Many people who later develop alcoholism begin drinking for the same social, psychological and cultural factors as their non-alcoholic friend. People drink for a variety of reasons: to feel more comfortable in social situations, to feel a part of their peer group, to laugh and forget their troubles and so on. Drinkers learn through experience how much alcohol they can 'handle" and which alcoholic beverages they prefer. They enjoy the stimulating effects and social camaraderie drinking can seems to help produce. Freud said that it is human nature to seek pleasure and avoid pain. This process functions to sustain us as human beings, and motivates us to strive to fulfill our survival needs for food, shelter, and propagation.

People repeat actions that produce pleasure or reward. Freud has referred to this as a kind of "organic elasticity".[49] The drinker wants to return to an earlier time when a state of pleasure or lack of pain was present, and seeks to re-create that pleasurable past. Many an alcoholic will try to recapture the blissful feelings of the moment when he or she first began to drink. "Evidence has shown that alcohol and other drugs of abuse (AOD's) are chemical surrogates of such natural reinforcers".[50] The alcoholic drinks more and more in a vain attempt to escape his/her problems or pain only to find serious problems piling up all around him. A growing sense of despair leads to yet more drinking, and the cycle continues. Alcoholics who continue to drink can face life-reducing consequences, including institutionalization, incarceration, and premature death. Unless an alcoholic abstains from ingesting alcohol and arrests the physical aspect of the addiction, little can be done to help him or her.

Psychological, cultural, and social factors play a role in the alcoholic's drinking behaviors and patterns, but they do not determine whether he/she will become addicted to alcohol. Many factors contribute to this and more are being discovered, but the alcoholic's genetic make-up, hormones, brain chemistry and enzymes all play a role in the development of the disease. It is important for psychotherapists and physicians in the field of addiction to be open to these new forms of treatment based on the latest scientific discoveries if we are going to be able to reach a larger number of sick and suffering alcoholics and help them effectively.

Alcoholics are Metabolically Different

Sooner or later, the drinking patterns and behaviors of the alcoholic begin to change from that of their non-alcoholic friends and colleagues. The alcoholic starts drinking more and more and oftentimes displays a very high tolerance to alcohol. Once the alcoholic picks up the first drink it triggers a physical addiction coupled by a mental obsession. The person wants more and more alcohol to try to satisfy the intense craving that has been ignited.

Personality changes often occur and can be very strange and puzzling to the onlooker or loved one. Shy people can become very verbose and the "life of the party"; those once deemed timid can become argumentative and hostile; formerly caring types can turn cold and cruel. Whatever the manifestations, a personality change is involved that can be seen by those around them. As the early stages of alcoholism set in, the alcoholic becomes more and more self-centered, moody, depressed and isolated. These characteristics progress along with the disease. It is important to note that even though psychological, social and cultural factors influence the user, alcoholism the disease is activated only by drinking alcohol. It is the alcohol that triggers the addiction—a physical allergy as it were. If a person stops drinking, the disease is arrested.[51] If, however, the person continues to drink, the disease of alcoholism continues to progress.

The Role of Genetics in Alcoholism

The cause of alcoholism is a complex blend of genetic, physical, psychological, environmental, social, and spiritual factors that can vary greatly among affected individuals. Genetics plays a crucial role in the disease of alcoholism. Current research indicates that children of alcoholics are four to five times more likely to inherit alcoholism than those children born to non-alcoholic parents. It was known for more than a hundred years that alcoholism runs in families, but it was not until Dr. Donald Goodwin studied adopted children whose biological fathers were alcoholics that insights into the genetic link were gained.

Goodwin's research determined that sons of male alcoholics were four times more likely to inherit the disease. Even if these boys were adopted and raised in non-alcoholic homes the disease would still manifest itself, leading researchers to the genetic rather than environmental link to alcoholism. These boys were also more likely to develop the disease earlier in life (in their twenties).[52] Goodwin's studies postulated that alcoholics do not drink because they are lonely, angry, dissatisfied, or immature. Alcoholics drink because they have physically inherited a susceptibility to alcohol which results in addiction if and when they drink. Of the nation's 10 million alcoholics, half are thought to be genetically predisposed. The other half develops the disease over time, usually later in life, and many have anxiety disorders and phobias as well.[53]

Dr. Marc Schuckit of the University of California at San Diego, the chief researcher of the alcoholism unit at the Veterans Administration Hospital in La Jolla, explains that many genes are involved in inheriting alcoholism, so there are many ways to become an alcoholic. He likens the disease to diabetes. In such a case some people are born at risk genetically and are more likely to develop the disease depending on environment choices and lifestyles.

New research also indicates that alcoholics and social drinkers metabolize ethanol on different pathways. Dr. David Rutstein of Harvard Medical School recently found a substance, 2, 3-butanediol, in the blood stream of alcoholics that was not present in the social drinkers, further indicating the metabolic differences. P-3 waves are involved in the brain's ability to make decisions. Dr. Helen Neville of the Salk Institute in La Jolla and Dr. Henri Begleiter in Brooklyn found that P-3 waves in alcoholics after one drink are markedly different than those waves of a social drinker. In both groups the waves were the same before a drink was administered.

This new research has not yet explained how the disease is inherited and how it alters brain and body chemistry, but it is believed that someday science will have these answers, which will help doctors treat alcoholism more effectively in the future.

The Biology of Alcoholism

Even with all the new medical findings in the field of alcoholism, much is still unknown. Identifying the biological and behavioral effects of the disease is therefore more useful in understanding it than is seeking to strictly define it. Alcoholics are people who organize their lives around alcohol. They have a mental obsession coupled with a physical craving (addiction). The alcoholic will continue to drink even though the drinking causes increased difficulty in their personal and professional lives. They will continue to drink even if they lose the love of their family members. They will continue to drink even if they lose their jobs. They will continue to drink even if they lose their health. They will continue to drink even if they lose their lives. The stages of alcoholism are explored later in this chapter. Some of the biological effects are:

- Changes in the structure and composition of the membranes surrounding brain cells that dictate memory, emotions, and all bodily functions.

- An increasing dependence by the brain cells on alcohol for normal functioning.

- Symptoms of withdrawal when alcohol is not present in the brain.

- Acute damage to the central nervous system

- Increase in the neurotransmitters controlling brain communication.

- Potentially lethal damage to the liver, pancreas, heart and stomach, and an increased susceptibility to certain cancers.

- Impotence in males.

- Increases in psychological disorders like anxiety and phobias, and—especially among women—depression.

- Fetal Alcohol Syndrome (FAS), characterized by mental retardation, stunted growth, and facial disfigurations, in babies born to mothers who abuse alcohol during pregnancy.

- Blood abnormalities including anemia, reduced white cell counts, broken blood vessels and enlarged red cells. [54]

This list is by no means complete. The damage of alcoholism spreads throughout the individual's body and beyond. Alcoholism damages families, friends, communities, businesses, and the very fabric of a society.

Alcoholics are Chemically Different

Currently some 40 to 50 neurotransmitters have been discovered in the brain, but Dr. Floyd Bloom, a neurobiologist at the Scripps Clinic in La Jolla, California suggests that there is strong evidence to suggest that ten times as many may exist, and that these chemicals play a crucial role in how alcohol affects our bodies. Dr. Bloom believes "that alcohol influences processes by which neurotransmitters are released … and may inhibit some and promote others. It certainly alters known neurotransmitters in many ways in different parts of the brain." Ironically, scientists feel that maybe alcohol is not what makes people drunk but the by-products of alcohol which alter the neurotransmitters in the brain. One such group of by-products is called tetrahydroisoquinolines (TIQ's), which have been identified as chemically related to opiates. In light of this finding, Dr. Bloom suggests there may be a common mechanism for addiction.[55]

Another theory suggests that alcoholism is a deficiency in certain neurotransmitters, and that alcoholics are trying to correct this deficiency by drinking alcohol. A study at the UCLA Medical Center is currently underway to compare receptors in the brains of deceased alcoholics and non-alcoholics to see if this can be proven.[56]

Several researchers have suggested that acetaldehyde rather than alcohol itself is responsible for addiction. Acetaldehyde is the intermediate byproduct of alcohol metabolism and appears to be a major cause of alcoholic drinking. Dr. Charles Lieber, Chief of research at the Bronx Veterans Administration Hospital found that the same amount of alcohol produced very different levels of blood acetaldehyde in the bodies of alcoholics and non-alcoholics and that the breakdown into acetate was at about half the rate in non-alcoholics. This slowed down process in alcoholics is thought to be what cause the accumulation of acetaldehyde in their bodies.[57] This finding may answer the age-old question of whether an alcoholic drinks too much because his/her body is abnormal or is it abnormal because of heavy drinking.

According to this research the alcoholic has an abnormal bodily function in relation to processing alcohol. This liver enzyme malfunction triggers the alcoholic's need to drink more and more to counter the painful effects of the progressive build-up of acetaldehyde.[58]

As previously stated, endorphins are opiate-like substances produced and experienced in the brain as a "natural high". Endorphins decrease if a narcotic is taken into the body on a regular basis and the network of nerve cells called the locus coeruleus (LC) becomes dependent on the outside substance for its endorphin supply. If this is not met, a craving is set-up as the body reacts to the withdrawal of the opiate.[59]

Clonidine is a drug used for hypertension whose effects have recently been studied in lab rats. It has been found to lessen the withdrawal symptoms on the LC. It is hoped that this drug might also be helpful in easing other withdrawal symptoms from alcohol and cigarettes as well. Research is currently underway as to its effectiveness but the early results are promising.[60]

Alcoholism is a Three-Fold Disease

Chronic alcoholism is said to be a progressive three-fold disease. It is characterized by a physical addiction to the chemical alcohol, coupled by a mental obsession, and in its most extreme manifestation,—by what can be described as a spiritual bankruptcy or soul sickness.

The Physical Disease

The physical addiction, or allergy, to alcohol has a wide range of dramatic effects on the human body as more and more alcohol is ingested over a period of time. The addicted individual has an incessant craving for the substance alcohol, an increased tolerance for its effects, and progressive loss of control over it.

Often the early damage to the body is not obvious to the alcoholic or others, but as the alcoholism continues through excessive drinking, the damage becomes apparent to everyone.

As the physical addiction deepens, the person can experience a range of symptoms from fatigue and flu-like feelings when withdrawing from a binge or a hangover, to sweating, shaky hands, headache, and nausea, lack of mental clarity, agitation and depression. The more chronic symptoms experienced in late-stage alcoholism include memory black-outs, organ damage, compromised immunological resources leading to lowered resistance to other diseases, alcohol poisoning due to high levels of consumption, nutritional deficiencies, malnutrition, organ failure, chronic depression, suicidal ideation, susceptibility to certain cancers, liver disease, and ultimately, death. Only complete abstinence from alcohol will arrest the physical allergy and its effects. Alcoholism is treatable but not curable.

The Mental Disease

The mental addiction or obsession is characterized by an ever-growing preoccupation with alcohol and all the behaviors that go along with drinking. A sample of the worries occupying the problem drinker's mind includes, "How much money is there for "partying"? And, on any given day, "What time can I start drinking?" If the alcoholic is going out, he/she will want to know, "How much alcohol will there be there? "When will I be able to drink?" As the disease progresses, so does the mental obsession. It shifts into deeper justifications for drinking, plans for binge drinking, and strategies for hiding from others how much he/she is drinking, along with mechanisms for denying and deceiving those around them about their drinking. All this activity occurs within the maelstrom created by a increasing loss of control, mentally as well as physically, complicated by the terror of memory lapses, sensitivity to noises, deepening depression, desperation, paranoia, vague and often irrational fears, feelings of doom, and so on. At some point, the choice becomes whether to continue the decline or seek help trying to stop it.

The mental obsession with alcohol is best treated with psychotherapy after the abstinence from alcohol is established. The obsession, for some, can be a very difficult part of the recovery process. As we understand more about the addictive brain, and the role of brain chemistry in alcoholism, better treatment options will be developed. The support of a sponsor, a therapist, and the fellowship of a 12-step program are currently the best remedies for the addictive mind.

The Spiritual Disease

The spiritual or self-worth aspects of the disease begin with low self-esteem coupled with self-centeredness and self-centered fears. Alcoholics frequently suffer feelings of being separate, different, and isolated from their fellows. This chronic loneliness and depression has led to approximately 1/3 of all alcoholics committing suicide.[61] This soul sickness or spiritual bankruptcy is so painful that the addict will seek to medicate the feelings with alcohol, which offers temporary relief, at least in the early stages. Carl Jung writes of this spiritual emptiness when he says, "The craving for alcohol is the equivalent of a low level of the spiritual thirst of our being for wholeness; expressed in medieval language: the union with God."[62] Marion Woodman, a Jungian analyst points out, "they have displaced their search for spirit onto a material object (alcohol)." She believes that our addictive behavior is "an expression of a much deeper malaise: the millennia-old rejection of our bodies, our feelings ... and the endemic addiction to self-perfection". As the addict continues to drink, he/she loses more and more contact with his/her inner self, his/her relationships with others, and any concept of a higher power.[63] Famous writer F. Scott Fitzgerald believed that his alcoholism was the result of his fear and insecurity about his writing:

> I was afraid I wasn't good enough. Always had been afraid, but maybe in youth believed age would remedy it. Now I was middle-aged and afraid I'd never be good enough ... I had plenty of time to face myself now and survive, I had to take stock of whatever I was and get the courage to face it without trying to drown the image in drink again. I had to stop running away from myself, I had to stop hiding from myself, I had to stop drowning myself in gin ... I had been afraid to do my best for fear my best would not be good enough.[64]

Fitzgerald believed that he drank because of his fears about his writing ability, but medical research has proven over the last twenty-five years that emotional illness is often the result of alcoholic drinking and not necessarily the cause of it.

Alcoholics Anonymous (A.A.) believes that there are only 3 possible outcomes if an alcoholic continues to drink: the person will be incarcerated, committed to a hospital or mental institution, or will die prematurely. This is a very grim picture except for the fact that the disease can be arrested by total abstinence. A.A. is based on helping the alcoholic to achieve and maintain sobriety by addressing and supporting all three aspects of the disease.

4

A PROGRESSIVE DISEASE

The Three Stages of Alcoholism

First the man takes a drink
Then the drink takes a drink
Then the drink takes the man.

—Japanese proverb

James Milam and Katherine Ketcham, clinical psychologists and nationally known authorities in the field of alcoholism, outline three stages of the progression of alcoholism in their book, *Under the Influence.* They are the

1. Early, adaptive stage

2. Middle stage

3. Late, deteriorative stage (pp. 47–94)

What are the signs and significances of each stage and how do we identify the problem in our friend, loved one, co-worker, child, or in ourselves?

Alcoholism: Stage One (Early/Adaptive)

The "high" high is the elation felt by alcoholics in the early stages of the disease when the alcohol is doing for them what they were not able to do for themselves. Suddenly, the feelings of isolation disappear and they feel comfortable and confident in social situations. They feel relaxed and buoyant as never before. Low self esteem is replaced with self-assurance. They do not feel "sick" from drinking alcohol, on the contrary, they feel great. It is the magic elixir that they have been searching for all their lives. Alcohol is seen as the missing piece that allows them to feel whole. The early phases of alcoholism can be likened to those of a love affair, and the onlooker would be hard-pressed to convince the problem drinker that these were early warning signs of alcoholism. Slowly the alcoholic begins to notice that he/she drinks differently than his or her fellows. Surely they are the first to come to a party and the last to leave, but their friends 'just don't have what it takes—they are wimps'. Alcoholics often feel great pride in their ability to drink anyone under the table and boast about it as if it was some skill that they had learned, when in fact it is another symptom of early alcoholism. Tolerance is the result of physiological changes in the liver and the nervous system altering the brain's electrical impulses.

Another difference in the alcoholic as opposed to the non-alcoholic is the issue of performance. The alcoholic often performs and feels "better" while drinking, and the detrimental effects are felt only while not drinking, or while 'sobering up'. This is because of the blood alcohol level (BAL). As Milam & Ketcham point out, "To acquire the therapeutic effects, he must keep his BAL at a fairly constant level by continuing to drink; if he stops drinking, his BAL will drop and both psychological and physiological performance will rapidly deteriorate."[65] This dynamic sets the stage for maintenance drinking. Whether the alcoholic is consciously aware of it or not, she is attempting to manage her BAL, because if she doesn't, she will suffer the ever-worsening withdrawal effects of the dependency.

At this point, the addiction is already established, because in order to have the cells function normally they need to drink alcohol. This is why the alcoholic eventually loses control over his/her drinking. Larger amounts of alcohol will be needed and the dependence has taken hold to the point where ceasing to drink would cause negative withdrawal symptoms. It is ironic that the very thing that alcohol is used for in the beginning—to alleviate stress, fear, and feelings of isolation and despair—are later recreated in the form of alcohol withdrawal. This is the nightmare of the alcoholic, and the vicious cycle that leads to further and further deterioration. Once this dependence is established the alcoholic, even in the early stage, cannot return to social, non-alcoholic drinking. The analogy often used is that once a cucumber becomes a pickle, it cannot go back to being a cucumber again, although that is one of the great hopes of the alcoholic—that he/she can someday drink normally again. Well-known journalist William Seabrook writes of this in his book, *Asylum*, the account of his alcoholism and treatment at Bloomingdale Hospital in Westchester County in the 1930's. He writes, "To go out and never be able to touch a cocktail, glass or wine, or highball again would be a poor sort of cure, if it could be termed a cure at all. I said that I still hoped to be really "cured", cured so well that I would be able to take a highball with my friends …"[66]

Stage Two: Middle Phase

The process of drinking, suffering the effects of drinking, and then drinking again to stop the symptoms of drinking is an ever-downward spiral. The second stage of alcoholism is identified by three important features, as stated by Dr. Milam: "physical dependence is experienced in acute and protracted withdrawal syndromes of craving, and loss of control." As the alcoholic continues to drink heavily, the cells in the body have to adjust in order to process the alcohol. The cells adapt to living in an alcohol environment. The alcoholic will experience acute withdrawal syndrome upon ceasing to drink, and the subsequent withdrawal symptoms indicating the person's addiction may occur months or even years after the alcoholic has stopped drinking.[67] Feelings of depression, irritability, fear, anxiety, and uneasiness can plague a sober alcoholic for a long period of time—one of the reasons members of Alcoholics Anonymous insist on regular attendance at meetings long after sobriety is achieved. Without continued assistance with the emotional issues involved in alcoholism, the alcoholic can easily justify going back to drinking because he/she, ironically, can feel worse not drinking. This is one of the great ironies of alcoholism, and one that needs to be addressed by the individual if sobriety is to be maintained. The rule of thumb is that the more a person drinks, the more intense the suffering of early sobriety because of the damage done over time to the chemical and electrical functioning of the brain, blood, and organs, and so on, by alcohol. Withdrawal symptoms, therefore, can vary widely, but when a person reaches the second stage of alcoholism, the hangover symptoms can go from anxiety and free-floating fears, brownouts, confusion, shakiness, nausea, cold sweats, hyperactivity and/or lethargy, etc., to convulsions, black-out seizures, hallucinations, delirium tremors, malnutrition, deep feelings of shame and hopelessness, low blood sugar, and more. Delirium tremens (DT's) is Latin for "shaking insanity". This extremely terrifying withdrawal symptom speaks for itself. In her memoir, *Part of a Long Story,* Carlotta Monterey O'Neill recalls her life with famous playwright husband, Eugene O'Neill:

> O'Neill's later years were clouded by the near total collapse of his health. His tremor became so severe that he found it impossible to write after 1943. Friends purchased a Dictaphone for him, but it was hopeless.[68]

In the mid-1940's, O'Neil's depression and sense of hopelessness is best expressed when he wrote this inscription for his tombstone:

Eugene O'Neil
There Is Something
To Be Said
For Being Dead

This great talent was, in the end, unable to write or to appreciate any part of life. Anyone who has experienced the second/third stage of alcoholism can relate to his words to one extent or another.

Alcohol has been referred to as the great robber. If an alcoholic continues to drink, the alcohol will rob that person of all his or her material possessions, all talents and wisdom, all loved ones. Eventually it will rob the alcoholic of himself or herself. Hemingway, another famous American writer plagued not only by alcoholism but by a chronic depression which led to his suicide in 1961, often used his characters to speak for him in his battle with addiction. In his book, *For Whom the Bell Tolls,* his character, Jordon, speaks of his addiction to absinthe and how it robbed him of everything he held dear:

> One cup of it took the place of the evening papers, of all the old evenings in cafes, of all chestnut trees that would bloom now in this month, of the great slow horses of the outer boulevards, of book shops, of kiosques, of galleries, of the Parc Mountsouris, of the Stade Buffalo, and the Butte Charmont ... and of being able to read and relax in the evening; of all the things he had enjoyed and forgotten and that came back to him when he tasted that opaque, bitter, tongue-numbing, brain-warming, stomach-warming, idea-changing liquid alchemy.

Craving a drink quickly turns from wanting a drink in the early stages because it feels so good, to needing a drink in stage two to stave off the effects of withdrawal. Milam & Ketcham point out, "As tolerance increases and physical dependence sets in, the alcoholic loses psychological control over his physiological need for alcohol. It is at this point that the alcoholic loses the ability to say, "no" to a drink and alcohol becomes the driving force in the alcoholic's life. Nothing stands in the way of a drink from that point on. The alcoholic has lost control of his drinking and will never regain control again. There can be temporary attempts at regaining control, but it is only a matter of time before the alcoholic is drinking at the same level (or worse) than before. The destructive effects of alcoholism are clearly and poignantly described by author Charles O.Gorham in his novel, *Wine of Life*:

One thing about alcohol, it works. It may destroy a man's career, ruin his marriage, turn him into a zombie unconscious in a hallway—but it works. In the short term, it works much faster than a psychiatrist or a priest or the love of a husband or a wife. Those things take time. They must be developed ... but alcohol is always ready to go to work at once. Then, minutes, half an hour, the little formless fears are gone or turned back into harmless amusement. But they come back. Oh yes, and they bring reinforcements. [69]

Stage Three: The Final Phase

When you get to the point where you don't care whether you live or die—as I did—it's hard to believe in yourself again—you have slain a part of yourself. [70]

The image of the skid row bum, the derelict who has lost everything: his health, home, job self-respect—but who is still drinking—is what most people think of as an alcoholic. In fact, this person has been an alcoholic for quite some time and this is the final stage of alcoholism. Not every alcoholic in the final stage is a skid row bum, but every skid row bum drinking out of a paper bag is an alcoholic.

The final stage of alcoholism is the chronic, deadly stage where the person's mental and physical health is at risk. Alcohol is now a poison. Organ damage, malnutrition, mental confusion, all worsen, and death is on the horizon in one form or another. Suicides, accidents, cancer, liver disease, heart failure, pneumonia, pancreatitis, gastrointentestinal disease, are often what show up—on the alcoholic's death certificate as "cause of death" but alcoholism is the real culprit. It is unbelievable that only 14% of the deaths caused by alcoholism are so labeled. [71] If every alcoholic who died of alcoholism was labeled as such on his/her death certificate, society would place alcoholism as perhaps the Number One killer of Americans.

Differences Between Male and Female Alcoholics

It has been only recently that medicine has begun to seriously focus on the differences between men and women at a genetic level. Researchers are now discovering how different men and women truly are from one another. Women are different in their bone structure, immune systems, and hormones, as well as in their reproductive functions. Researchers have shown that every cell in the human body is encoded with gender, and biochemical variations are rooted in its genetic structure. [72] Men and women respond to prescribed medications differently, for example, and therefore, doctors need to determine dosage not just by age but also by gender. Dr. Mark Saralyn, endocrinologist at Yale Hospital and senior medical advisor to NASA observes, "Despite mounting evidence showing men and women responding differently to the same drug, most physicians' and their patients are still not aware that gender matters when prescribing medications." Eight of the ten medications taken off the market in a five year period were removed because they were particularly dangerous to women.[73]

In 1993, Congress mandated that clinical trials include women. Prior to this, medical models were based on research conducted only on males. Fortunately, now, all of that is changing, and doctors such as Denise L Faustman, M.D., Ph.D., associate professor of medicine at Harvard Medical School, are discovering that the 'one size fits all' medicine is inadequate, and that sex-based biological research needs to replace the old model.

This is beginning to have an impact on the disease of alcoholism and the field of addiction as well. Women, for example, suffer more from depression than men (due in part to less serotonin production), and have a harder time quitting smoking (along with being twice as likely to develop lung cancer). Women have less body water than men and therefore achieve higher concentrations of alcohol in the blood. They also sustain more acute liver damage from alcohol (due in part to a higher fat content in the body). Also, an important enzyme, alcohol dehydrogenase, key in metabolizing alcohol in the body, works differently in men than it does in women. In men, it breaks down much of the alcohol in the stomach so that less alcohol enters the circulatory system. Because this enzyme is less active in females, more alcohol is allowed to enter into their bloodstreams.[74] (NIAA Alcohol Alert #10, 1994) Men get more relief from drugs such as Advil, whereas women respond better to Kappa opioids that are traditionally used by the dentist.[75]

White males are at higher risk for alcohol abuse than women, although Native Americans still remain at the highest risk level. Hispanics, Asians and Blacks are still at a lower risk, according to a 2001–2002 survey by the National Epidemiologic Survey on Alcohol and related Conditions (NESARC). In the last decade the prevalence for alcohol dependence remained almost the same for men, but it increased for women, narrowing the gender gap. (NESARC Survey 2001–02)

Alcohol and the Unborn Child

Fetal Alcoholic Syndrome (FAS) was first identified in 1970 when the medical community realized that alcohol in the bloodstream of the mother can be toxic to the developing fetus. The symptoms vary and are affected by the amount of alcohol consumed and the trimester in which the alcohol is ingested. FAS is irreversible and tragic. The symptoms of FAS range from behavioral problems, disfigurement, stunted growth, learning problems to mental retardation and beyond.[76] When such a child is born, he/she may experience withdrawal symptoms not unlike those of a child born to a heroine or crack addict. These babies are, in fact, already alcoholics. In *The Biology of Alcoholism,* the researcher writes:

The alcoholic mother who has been drinking heavily through pregnancy, and particularly that mother who has actually had acute alcoholic withdrawal during pregnancy may have ingested sufficient alcohol to have developed incipient signs and symptoms of tolerance and physical dependence in the newborn child ... Such a child, in addition to having the hypothesized genetic propensity toward alcoholism has probably been exposed to high levels of alcohol during his intrauterine development. Such a child may actually have developed some level of tolerance and physical dependence during pregnancy and may be born-in a manner similar to that of children of heroine addicts—in an acute alcoholic withdrawal state.[77]

Fetal Alcohol Syndrome (FAS) is a 100% preventable disorder. Alcohol in a pregnant women's bloodstream can be toxic to the unborn child, especially during certain stages of development. What happens when a pregnant woman drinks? Within minutes of taking a drink the fetus takes the same drink. Alcohol is one of the leading causes of mental retardation in the Western world.[78] You don't have to be an alcoholic to hurt your unborn child, timing is a key factor. Ann Streissguth, one of the University of Washington's team of researchers that first identified the syndrome points out, "A really dangerous time is before you know that you are pregnant, so the best recommendation is to not drink when planning a pregnancy." It is believed that as few as one or two drinks a day, or four or five at a time can have an effect on the unborn child.[79]

It is believed that there is also a link between Attention Deficit Hypertension Disorder (ADHD) and drinking during pregnancy. Streissguth concludes, "The research is so meager ... FAS youngsters have troubling paying attention and thinking abstractly. They could be a huge population."

Alcohol and the Elderly

The number of alcoholics is expected to triple as baby boomers reach 50 years and older in the next fifteen years. Ron Hunsicker of the National Association of Addiction Treatment Providers states, "We need to prepare to meet the needs of older addicts." In a federal report in 1989 it was estimated that ten million older adults were at risk of suffering drug addiction—primarily to sleeping pills and tranquilizers. Linda Dreblow, MSW, who manages an older-adult program at Scripps Memorial Hospital McDonald Center in La Jolla, California states, "Older adults have fewer social contacts as time goes on, and a lack of knowledge about chemical dependency makes it harder for others to pick up on."[80] Withdrawal symptoms from these drugs can include shakiness, stomach upset, sleeplessness, confusion, irritability, and depression. Many times the withdrawal symptoms from these drugs cause the very symptoms that the patient was seeking to combat.

Risk Factors for older adults include:

- anxiety and/or depression due to illness or loss.
- diminished self esteem
- loss of a spouse or close friends
- loss of home and/or family
- overdosing on medications due to forgetfulness or not realizing generic brand similarities.
- taking dosages that are the same as for younger adults, which in fact may be too much. Doctors need to take age into consideration more when estimating dosages.
- Using more than one doctor for prescriptions because of various ailments.
- isolation and lack of communication
- alcohol use along with the medication

Many older adults do not realize that alcohol is a drug as well. Older alcoholics are divided into two categories: early-onset and late-onset drinkers. According to Smithers Alcoholism Rehabilitation Center in New York City, approximately 2/3 of the older alcoholics are early-onset drinkers. They have abused alcohol for most of their lives, and often have multiple health issues in old age as a result. The remaining 1/3 are late-onset alcoholics, age 60+, who have developed the problem later in life and therefore have a better chance of recovery. Renee Zito, of the Smithers facility, notes that, "with abstinence, proper diet and time, recovery can be complete." The late-onset drinkers usually began drinking heavily as the result of a trauma or deep personal loss. Addressing these issues is also an important component for recovery. Dr. Larry W. Dupree, clinical psychologist and associate research professor in the department of Aging and Mental Health at the Florida Institute, University of South Florida, Tampa gives us a list of things to look for if we suspect an older person of alcohol or drug abuse. Any of these warning signs are important to follow up on.

Symptoms to look for in older adults:

- Abrupt or significant changes in behavior: hostility, paranoia.
- Forgetfulness, unsteady gait, slurred speech, or trembling hands.
- Previously controlled (via medication) conditions now out of control (e.g., diabetes, hypertension).
- Complaints of insomnia; frequent napping; absence of restful sleep.
- Deterioration in grooming, housekeeping and eating habits.
- Bottles stashed in the home (alcohol or pill).
- Falls, broken bones, bruises or burns.[81]

It is often very difficult to confront older people about their addiction because, like younger people, they often don't think they have this problem. The older population is also carrying the stigma of alcoholism from their upbringing. The American Medical Association did not introduce the disease concept of alcoholism until 1956. Older people grew up thinking of alcoholics as skid row bums who were morally weak and deranged. Educating them is an important part to being able to help them with their addiction. As Dr. LeClair, the founder of Smithers and a recovering alcoholic for nearly forty years says: 'There are no long-term chemical answers to life." (*Addiction*, 1999, p. 322)

In light of all the new research it seems obvious that gender-based biology will be a key component in determining more effective ways to treat addiction in men, women, boys, girls and the elderly, because each group has very specific differences, and therefore, different treatment needs.

Alcohol and Depression

Women are twice as likely to suffer from depression as men. This is partially due to lower serotonin production in females. The National Institute of Mental Health (NIMH) estimates approximately 12 million women and 6 million men in any given year are suffering from depressive illness. Fewer than half those suffering actually seek treatment, even though 80% of those seeking help do improve. Men are much more likely to seek help and/or recognize that they are in fact depressed. Depression can be caused by many factors including: Postpartum depression (PPD), which affects 10–20% of new mothers; Seasonal Affect Disorder (SAD) which is cause in part by reduced sunlight in winter and increased melatonin production due to the winter's darkness; Post Traumatic Stress Disorder (PTSD) caused by a severe trauma; according to NIMH 2.5 million Americans suffer from Bipolar Disorder (BPD) (more than half BPD sufferers have a chemical dependency problem as well); brain injury; other mental illnesses and alcoholism (alcoholics are nearly twice as likely to suffer from depression). (Rowner, 2004, pp. 2–4)/lost reference?

Howard University professor, Yousef Tizabi and his colleagues studied rats as a model for depression after observing that many depressed people who smoked cigarettes experienced more difficulty quitting than people who were not depressed. Tizabi deduced that the habit may be the subconscious effort to self-medicate through nicotine. In his study the rats were given mecamylamine, a nicotine receptor antagonist, to block the beneficial properties of nicotine. The rats were then no longer interested in getting the nicotine. This may prove an important tool in the future for treating nicotine addiction.

According to the National Institute of Mental Health (NIMH), symptoms of depression include; a persistent, sad, anxious or empty feeling; hopelessness, pessimism, worthlessness, shame, low self esteem, social withdrawal and lack of interest, loss of interest in hobbies, activities, grooming and self care, decreased energy, sleeping difficulties, difficulty concentrating or making decisions or planning; physical symptoms can include; headaches, digestive problems, eating problems, chronic pain, suicide attempts or thoughts of suicide. These symptoms can be found in individuals in varying degrees from mild to severe. Major Depressive Disorder (MDD) is in evidence when the depression is severe enough to interfere with regular daily functioning. It can occur once or re-occur throughout one's lifetime.

Scientists at Washington University believe that they have identified a specific gene associated with depression and alcoholism. This discovery was noted in the September 6, 2004 in the issue of the Journal for Human Molecular Genetics. The team reported analyzing samples of DNA from 2,310 people representing 262 families in which at least three of the family members were alcoholics. The researchers found a region in Chromosome 7 that looked very similar in the alcoholics. The scientists then studied the region of Chromosome 7 in people depressed but not necessarily alcoholic, and the similarity was also present. In conclusion, the group that was depressed and alcoholic were the most likely to have this similarity in Chromosome 7. Once the gene region in Chromosome 7 was identified, the researchers were then able to identify the gene CHRM2, one that is related to a type of cellular receptor involved in many varying brain functions, including attention, learning memory and cognition. This finding will hopefully open the way for further understanding of alcohol and depression, and could lead to more effective treatment and diagnosis.[82]

5

MYTHS AND STIGMAS

A History of the Treatment of Alcoholism

It is important to understand the history of the treatment of alcoholism and the ways in which society has viewed the alcoholic in order to fully understand the myths and stigmas associated with the disease, and why it has taken so long to change public perceptions. The American Medical Association's recognition of alcoholism as a disease in 1956 paved the way for studying its effects on the entire body, physical as well as psychological, but attitudes about the illness and its treatments have changed slowly. The physical and psychological components of alcoholism are inextricably linked, and complete recovery can be achieved only when both aspects of the disease are fully treated.

The Identification of Alcoholism as a Disease

In 1804, Thomas Trotter, an Edinburgh physician, wrote a paper stating his belief that alcoholism was indeed a disease:

> I consider drunkenness, strictly speaking, to be a disease produced by a remote cause, and giving birth to actions and movements in the living body that dis-order the functions of health.

Trotter's essay provoked a controversy, the divisiveness of which continues even today. His essay asked society to ponder the question: Is alcoholism prima-rily a physiological disease, or is it a symptom of character inadequacy and emo-tional weakness? This is still the root source of conflict and confusion in the alcoholism field today. Images of the skid-row bum or the street junkie stereotyp-ically portray the addict as immutably flawed in character, and even depraved. This attitude is understandable when we study the damage that second- and third- stage alcoholism can cause in the individual's character and brain function.

Bill Wilson, founder of Alcoholics Anonymous writes of his drinking experience, "I had been at the gates of insanity ... and other people were obliterated by the intensity of my narcissism." At the stage of addiction Wilson describes, not a single other basic human need is more important than getting the next drink—not food, not water, not even the respect of loved ones. Under that seemingly self-imposed level of neediness, it is easy to understand why society has judged the sick and suffering alcoholic so harshly. The alcoholic was considered a sinful and pitiful creature responsible for his own many troubles. If, however, excessive drinking were to be seen as a disease, as Trotter held it is, then perhaps the drinker cannot be held responsible for his own actions. The question then emerges of whether considering alcoholism a disease protects the alcoholic from moral condemnation and judgment. On the contrary, members of the medical profession were upset by Trotter's essay, as physicians had been limited at that time to treating the physical complications of excessive drinking and doing so with a mixture of fear and disgust. Further questions were anything but sympathetic to sufferers of this newly identified illness, including: How does one come to suffer such a disease? How is it contracted?

In 1841, the Washington Home in Boston opened as an institution for inebriates, helping to launch a 60-year period of expanding awareness of alcoholism and treatment centers. In 1870, the American Association for the Cure of Inebriates opened as well, one of many established at that time across the United States. Despite the slowly growing research about alcoholism these centers helped to foster, however, the understanding that it was a disease was not generally accepted among the populace.

Although the 1919 Volstead Act established national prohibition and reduced total alcohol consumption in this country, it had little effect on alcoholism. The Act was a misguided attempt to legislate morality and was repealed on December 5, 1933.

The wellspring of the recovery movement began in the 1920's and 30's in part by a Christian evangelical organization known as the Oxford Group. The name came from the early meetings that were held in Oxford, England. Also known as the First Century Christian Fellowship or "the fellowship", it functioned as a non-denominational, charismatic, prayer and healing group founded by ex-Lutheran minister Frank Buchman (1878–1961). Buchman's teaching consisted of the "Five C's"—Confidence, Conviction, Confession, Conversion, and Continuance. This structure and practice would later embody the Twelve Step Recovery program of Alcoholics Anonymous organized by Bill Wilson and Dr. Bob Smith in Akron, Ohio, in 1934. Meanwhile, halfway around the world in Zurich, Switzerland, a wealthy American named Rowland H. placed himself in 1931 in the care of Dr. Carl Jung for almost a year to treat his chronic drinking problem. Rowland relapsed shortly after his initial treatment and returned to Jung for more advice. Jung was blunt and to the point, and told Rowland that medicine and psychiatry could not help him. Nothing short of "a general conversion" or spiritual experience would help him. Jung knew from his experience that the body and the mind could not heal if the soul was sick. At this point, medicine regarded alcoholism as a personality disorder demonstrated through a lack of character and will-power. Jung's theory contradicted all of that when he wrote:

> Among all of my patients in the second half of life—that is to say, over thirty-five—there has not been one whose problem in the last resort was not that of finding a religious outlook on life. It is safe to say that every one of them fell ill because he had lost that which the living religions of every age have given to their followers, and none of them has really been healed who did not regain his religious outlook.[83]

Rowland returned to the United States and joined the Oxford Group, where he was released from the compulsion to drink by a conversion experience. The Oxford Group stressed the importance of prayer and meditation and the confession of one's "sins". Rowland passed the message on to his friend, Ebby Thacher, who was then able to stay sober through his successful treatment via the Oxford Group. In the Autumn of 1933, Bill Wilson was admitted to Townes Hospital where he met Dr. Duncan Silkworth. Silkworth was the first person to tell Bill that he had a disease. Bill recalls:

> Dr. Silkworth had pronounced me hopeless … He told me that I was a victim of a neurotic compulsion to drink, that no amount of willpower, education, or treatment could check. He also added that I was the victim of a bodily derangement which might be in the nature of an allergy—a physical malfunction that virtually guaranteed brain damage, insanity or death.[84]

In November of 1934, old time friend Thacher came to Bill's house to carry the message of sobriety. Wilson wanted sobriety, but was put off by the heavy religiosity of the group and went back to drinking again. By December 11, 1934 Wilson was once again admitted to Townes Hospital. The several cans of beer that Bill drank on his way to the hospital would prove to be his last. After being de-toxed Bill fell into a very deep depression. In desperation and despite being an agnostic he prayed' "If there be a God, will He show Himself!" As Bill recalls:

The result was instant, electric, beyond description. The place seemed to light up, blinding white. I knew only ecstasy and seemed on a mountain. A great wind blew, enveloping and penetrating me. To me, it was not of air, but of Spirit. Blazing, there came the tremendous thought "You are a free man." Then the ecstasy subsided. Still on the bed, I now found myself in a new world of consciousness which was suffused by a Presence. One with the Universe, a great peace stole over me. I thought, 'So this is the God of the preachers, this is the Great Reality.[85]

Bill Wilson from that point on was forever changed. He read William James' book "Varieties of Religious Experience" and was comforted by his wise words, "Conversion does alter motivation, and does semi-automatically enable a person to be and to do the formerly impossible". From that day forward Bill Wilson was not only able to stay sober, but he had the vision and the fortitude to be the co-founder of Alcoholics Anonymous. A.A. is thought by many to be the greatest spiritual movement of our time. Bill Wilson worked tirelessly with alcoholics until his death on January 24, 1971.

In May of 1935 Wilson was on a business trip in Akron, Ohio when he was tempted by the laughter in the hotel bar. He went to the lobby phone booth and looked up the church directory and called. He asked the minister if he knew any hopeless alcoholics he could talk to and the minister referred him to Dr. Bob Smith, an alcoholic physician. On Mother's Day, 1935 the two met for the first time. On June 10, 1935, Dr. Bob had his last drink and he never took another drink again right through to the day of his death. The seeds of Alcoholics Anonymous had been planted in 1935, on Mother's Day.

The Fellowship of Alcoholics Anonymous (A.A.) was founded by two ordinary men who had been given up as "hopeless" drunkards by their physicians. Bill Wilson and Dr. Bob Smith went on to set up a recovery program which has helped millions of alcoholics recover from alcoholism. A.A. demonstrated for the first time that alcoholics in significant numbers could recover and return to productive, useful lives. Most importantly, it proved that alcoholics, when they stayed sober, were decent, productive human beings and not hopeless degenerates.

Marty Mann, one of the first women members of Alcoholics Anonymous (A.A.), founded what was later to become the National Council on Alcoholism (NCA). Along with A.A., the NCA helped spread the idea that alcoholism is a treatable disease. This forced the church and the medical profession to modify their positions.

In 1956, the American Medical Association (AMA) finally declared alcoholism a physical disease. It was, however, still viewed by medical professionals as a self-inflicted symptom of an underlying psychological inadequacy.

The Weaknesses in Alcoholism Treatment

On the whole, major health professionals and hospitals are still unable to provide truly effective help for alcoholics. At a seminar on alcoholism sponsored by Interface in Boston in 1989, some were shocked to hear that in-patient facilities and detoxification centers have an 85% failure rate in the treatment of alcoholism. The failure rate is determined by a patient's continued sobriety for a period of one year. Milam & Ketchum believe that this low rate of recovery stems from the frequent treatment of alcoholism as primarily a psychological problem rather than a physical disease and systemic addiction. This is viewed more and more as a basic weakness of traditional treatments of alcoholism. Facilities following standard psychopathological treatment models typically underestimate the long-term effects of toxicity, malnutrition, hypoglycemia, and even withdrawal syndromes in causing or aggravating the alcoholic's psychological problems. Instead, these problems are perceived as arising from the inadequacy, depressiveness, anxiety, and self-destructive nature of the alcoholic. This view from society and the medical profession increases the alcoholic's guilt and shame.

Physicians in the past have received little or no medical training in alcoholism, and most did not have the experience or skill in recognizing or diagnosing alcoholism in its early stages. Not surprisingly, the majority had little or no familiarity with the available treatment methods of Alcoholics Anonymous' Twelve steps, or with up-to-date scientific literature. Again, the primary reason for this neglect is that the medical profession, along with the rest of society, historically classified alcoholism as a psychological disorder. Milam & Ketcham stated unequivocally:

> Both scientists and treatment professionals striving to advance the disease concept of alcoholism defeat their own aims by continuing to believe, or condoning the belief, that alcoholism is caused by heavy drinking, which in turn is caused by defects in the drinker's psychological, social, and cultural fabric. This is the belief that keeps alive all the age-old myths and misconceptions and the stigma, shame, and contempt for the alcoholic that continue to cloud the field of alcoholism. [86]

Psychiatrists virtually controlled the alcoholism field for many years. In the past ten years, however, that authority has come under attack. Psychiatrists have, in fact, been gradually phased out of federal alcoholism programs. The funds are now being given to biological and neuro-physiological disease researchers. The new leaders in the field, such as, Joan Borysenko, Ph.D., and Jacquelyn Small, Ph.D., are influenced by the abundance of research showing alcoholism as a physiological disease. Psychiatrists concentrating instead on the superficial psychological symptoms may even harm the patient by delaying treatment, increasing guilt and shame, and allowing the patient either to deny his or her drinking problem or blame it on someone or something else.

Underlying the revolt against psychiatric treatment of alcoholism is the accumulation of evidence that it simply does not work. In a survey of members of the Southern California Psychiatric Association, over one half of the psychiatrists who treated alcoholics reported no success with their patients, while the remainder had only 10% success. Once psychiatrists understand the physiological bases of the disease, their role will change. This has been demonstrated dramatically in the pioneering efforts of individual psychiatrists such as M. Scott Peck, David Ohlms, Peter Bourne, and Joseph Pursch.

Dr. M. Scott Peck, author and psychiatrist, discusses in his book, "Further Along the Road Less Traveled", the disturbing assertion that even today, psychiatrists practicing or studying alcoholism believe AA serves as a substitute for the addict's addiction. In fact, Scott believes that it is only about 1.5% of the reason for AA's effectiveness. He explains:

> When I was in psychiatry training thirty years ago, psychiatrists already knew that AA had a much better track record in working with alcoholics ... We believed that alcoholics had what we called "oral personality disorder" and that rather than opening their mouths to drink, they would get together at AA meetings and yap a lot and drink lots of coffee and smoke a lot of cigarettes ... and that would satisfy their oral needs.[87] 54

This stilted and condescending attitude among some professionals has not helped the alcoholic, his/her family, or society as a whole to respect the complexities of the disease. It is only when we can cast aside the conventional prejudices that real understanding and compassion can come forth. As Henry David Thoreau pointed out so aptly in his book, Walden, "It is never too late to give up your prejudices." A better understanding of the neuropsychological mechanisms in the brain, as well as new discoveries in genetics and gender-based medicine offer us new insights into the complexities of the disease of alcoholism effective treatment approaches. Perhaps through the lens of science we will finally be able to see the recovery potential of the alcoholic in a more realistic and favorable light.

Weaknesses in Treatment of Alcoholism in the Legal System

The whole approach to alcoholism by the legal system needs analysis and quite possibly, transformation. The alcohol and drug problem in this country is everybody's problem because it affects all members of our society. Government studies in recent years by the National Institute on Alcohol Abuse and Alcoholism (NIAAA), show clear causal relationships between alcohol and crime, including homicides, spousal abuse, and sexual offenses. In 1999, 30 % of the driving fatalities were caused by drunk driving, claiming an estimated 15,000 lives.[88] Generally, approximately 6 million people arrested in any given year are under the influence of drugs or alcohol at the time of their arrest, with average costs to society of $62 billion annually.[89]

These statistics endorse action by the criminal justice system to require effective alcoholism treatment to qualify for parole or probation, in addition to stiff sentences for alcohol-related crimes. Treatment should also be included with fines and/or sentences for minors adjudicated in alcohol-related legal issues as this can often present as a symptom of early alcoholism rather than mere psychological problems. According to Lee P. Brown, Ph.D., director of the Office of National Drug Control Policy, "A California study showed that for every dollar spent on treatment, seven dollars are returned to society, largely in the form of reduced spending on crime and health care." An extraordinary savings, not just financially, but in terms of the conservation of life and limb as well.

In recent years "safe driving" programs have been set up such as the Alcohol Safety Action Project (A.S.A.P.), Driving While Intoxicated (D.W.I.) and Driving Under the Influence (D.U.I.) Many AA committees cooperate with these programs and offer attendees an opportunity to learn about AA. Judges and probation officers, more than ever, rule that alcohol-related offenders attend AA as part of their sentence and/or probation requirements. Many of those attending AA meetings have gone on to become such members of AA and maintain sobriety. AA meetings are in many prisons thanks to the request in 1942 of Warden Clinton T. Duffy. He was the first warden to ask AA to hold meetings with inmates in San Quentin. Now AA meetings are held in prisons all over the country.

As science uncovers more and more facts about the disease of alcoholism and the role it plays in violent crimes, more programs and cooperation will develop among law enforcement agencies and treatment facilities. (Cooperating with the Court, AA Guidelines)

Strengths of Current Alcoholism Treatment Programs

Alcoholics Anonymous (A.A.), a world-wide organization, has saved millions of alcoholics, as well as spurring comprehensive research in the field of addiction and addiction treatment. Its members span 141 countries, and its numbers across the globe are growing. A.A.'s twelve steps has also spun off other addiction-based programs, such as Narcotics Anonymous, Gamblers/Debtors Anonymous, Overeaters Anonymous, Sexual Addiction Anonymous and the family support group Adult Children of Alcoholics (A.C.O.A.) and Co-dependency.

According to a 1994 Newsweek article, there are over 15 million+ people in 500,000+ self-help groups in the United States alone. "We used to hide under the bottle", says a member of A.A. in Moscow. "Now we have something to live for." There are more than 97,000 groups of Alcoholics Anonymous in the world. The success of AA is in the numbers, and a study of them shows the diversity of those willing to take the steps to sobriety. A 2001 survey of 7,500 members in the US and Canada conducted by the General Service Office of Alcoholics Anonymous found that

- 88% of the members were white,
- 5% Black,
- 4% Hispanic
- 2% Native American
- 1% Asian/other.

Of this group 33% were women and 67% men. The average age of an AA member was 46 years old and the age breakdown was:

- 2% under 21
- 9% age 21–30
- 24% 31–40

- 31% 41–50
- 20% 51–60
- 10% 61–70
- 4% were over 70. (AA Membership Survey, 2001)

Encouraging news was that 64% of the members received some type of treatment and/or counseling, and 73% of the members' physicians know they are in AA. Moreover, 38% were referred to AA by a healthcare professional. Significantly, 74% of the members who received treatment and/or counseling said it played an important role in directing them to AA. This illustrates the importance of supportive and well trained professionals in the treatment of this disease.

The average length of sobriety among those interviewed was seven years and the comparative duration of sobriety was reported as

- 48% sober more than 5 years
- 22% sober 1–5 years
- 30% sober less than one year.

Every three years a survey such as this one is conducted to provide information to the public as well as the professional community.[90]

6

SURVIVING ALCOHOLISM

Stages of Recovery

This recovery model emerged, in part, from Julie Bowden and Herbert Gravitz's stages of recovery outlined in their learning publication, "A Recovery Guide For Adult Children of Alcoholics". In it, the authors state that recovery occurs in predictable stages. These stages are the same whether you are the alcoholic or the child of an alcoholic. In my 25 years of working with alcoholics and their families I have modified Bowden and Gravitz's work to three predictable stages of recovery:

The Survivor Stage

Many alcoholics are caught in this stage. Drinking has shifted from being pleasure-driven to being need-driven to escape the pains of withdrawal. They need to drink to avoid feeling sicker than they already feel. As these alcoholics move from stage two to stage three of alcoholism, the symptoms of withdrawal worsen. Alcoholics in the later stages of alcoholism, experience seizures, DTs, and intense self-recrimination if they stop drinking. In the face of these known risks, therefore, denial serves as a mechanism for staving off the pain of withdrawal and continuing in the use of alcohol. The whole family can be in the grips of denial as well. Spouses denying their partner's alcoholism, children unable to admit their parents' addictions, episodes of abusive behavior and/or dysfunctional attitudes are all common during the survivor stage. Although the survivor stage is the first stage of the recovery process, recovery does not actually begin until the identification stage.

The Identification Stage

The Identification stage begins the moment the alcoholic or addict shifts from a refusal to acknowledge his/her alcohol abuse to a more realistic acceptance of her addiction. Alcoholism involves the acknowledgement and acceptance of the disease. This is also in line with the first step in the 12-step program, which states: "We admitted we were powerless over alcohol, and our lives had become unmanageable."

This stage involves admitting oneself as being alcoholic and realizing that one's claim to willpower had been grossly misstated. Accepting a more honest relationship with reality can be a liberating experience. It can also be frightening and humbling. The identification stage also involves a more realistic assessment of the past.

The Core Issue Stage

Bowden's next stage is called the Core Issue stage. This stage involves an active exploration of the ways that our refusal to admit powerlessness and our fear of being out of control affects our lives. Recovery is a continuous process of acknowledging the more realistic limits of willpower and the role that delusion and denial have played in perpetuating the disease. Core issues are rooted in our identity and they motivate all that we do. It is important to uncover these core beliefs if a personality change is to take place. AA does not blame the alcoholic for having the disease but it does demand that the sober alcoholic take responsibility for it, fulfilling the meaning of Emerson's concept of "self-reliance", wherein we take responsibility for our lives, grow up, hold ourselves accountable, and tell the truth. This is the basis for the amends steps in AA: Step Four: "Made a searching and fearless moral inventory"; and Steps 8–10, which involve amends or to 'make right". Step 8 states "Made a list of all persons we had harmed, and became willing to make amends to them all"; while Step 9 states: "made direct amends whenever possible, except when to do so would injure them or others", and Step 10: "continued to take personal inventory and when we were wrong, promptly admitted it".

Working through the steps with a sponsor brings about the healing of the distorted perceptions of the alcoholic. A sponsor is someone in the program who has already been through the steps and is there to guide the newcomer as he/she heals their unhealthy and self-defeating behaviors and attitudes. Understanding one's core beliefs and making amends for harmful and hurtful behavior to others while drinking is a very important part of the alcoholic's emotional healing. But it is not a small task, and this is why AA says that it is not for the person who needs it, it is for the person who wants it. This concept is reminiscent of John Calvin's sermon in 1536: the same sermon is addressed to a hundred persons, twenty receive it with the obedience of faith; the others despise, or ridicule, or reject, or condemn it. Only to a select minority would it seem about right. If a recovering alcoholic is among the lucky few who want recovery, he/she must guard it with his/her life, for there is nothing more precious to an alcoholic.

Treating the Physical Disease of Alcoholism

Genetic, brain, and biological research is proving in a more concrete way that alcoholism is a physical disease with emotional and spiritual components. The allergy to alcohol and the need to abstain from ingesting alcohol in any form must be recognized if the alcoholic is to be treated effectively. Arresting the physical trigger of the disease, as well as understanding the predisposing factors for the disease are essential if treatment is to be effective.

While psychological, cultural, and social factors definitely influence the alcoholic's drinking patterns and behavior, they have no effect on whether or not he/she becomes an alcoholic in the first place. Physiology, not psychology, determines whether one drinker becomes addicted to alcohol and another will not. Approximately 10% of all drinkers become alcoholics.[91] The alcoholic's enzymes, hormones, genes, and brain chemistry work together to create his/her abnormal reaction to alcohol.

Milam & Ketcham state that accumulated evidence clearly indicates that alcoholism is hereditary. Donald Goodwin, a Danish psychiatrist and researcher, has found clear evidence that alcoholism is passed on from parent to child through genes. He studied 5,000 cases from 1924–1947. In this blind study, Goodwin found that children of alcoholics have four times the risk of children of non-alcoholic biological parents of becoming alcoholic themselves even if they were separated from their parents at birth. Goodwin's studies provide compelling evidence that alcoholics do not drink addictively because they are depressed, immature, or dissatisfied. They drink addictively because they have inherited a physical susceptibility. Goodwin's study was supported by the National Association of Alcohol Abuse and Alcoholism.[92]

In the following case study Bruce's experience is aligned with the conclusions of Goodwin's study. Bruce was adopted at birth by non-drinking parents and raised in a stable, loving environment. Bruce developed alcoholism because he had inherited the disease from his birth parents:

Case Study:
Bruce C's Story

"Both My Biological Parents Were Active Alcoholics"

At this point in my sobriety I realize that I have a predisposition to alcoholism. I was adopted as an infant and did not know who my biological parents were until I was in my thirties. Both my biological parents were active alcoholics until the day they died in their late 80's. It was hard for me to understand this until I knew that a genetic link to alcoholism ran its course within me, even though I was raised by adoptive parents who were definitely not afflicted.

Today it doesn't matter how I got the disease. I have it and I actually now see it as a gift. I had always felt different as a child. I was a loner and felt like I didn't fit in with others. I would do silly things to try to impress kids and get them to like me, but this ploy rarely worked. I had a few friends, but I was always feeling lonely. There was always something missing and I didn't know what it was or how I could get it. It made me mad sometimes, and could make me act out. I would sabotage myself often. I would do really well at something until right at the last minute and then I would quit or wreck it. My thought was "I told you I wasn't good enough". It was self fulfilling prophecy. I pursued this cycle of self-defeat right into and through a drinking career.

When I was about thirteen or fourteen years old, I discovered pot and started smoking it regularly with my friends. Pot was a way to escape from the misery in which I found myself pretty much all the time. I had no interest in alcohol at that time, probably because I had seen what it did to people. At any rate, I was sure then I wanted no part of it. I was judging my insides by other people's outsides at that time anyway. I was letting outward appearances rule how I felt about things not only in my regular life, but when I came to see the effects of alcohol on people.

I was in college when I had my first real drunk, and I was hooked from the start. I loved the feeling. I finally understood why people who I had regarded as so messed up did what they did. It was wonderful: I could be whatever I wanted to be, say whatever I wanted to say—and I did. I had a 90-pound body and a 400-pound mouth, which got me in trouble from the get-go.

I always had people wanting to beat me up and sometimes they did. I didn't care. Alcohol was my best friend for a long time and I truly felt that if I just controlled it or drank the right varieties of it, I wouldn't get into trouble. I went through cycles of doing well, then getting into trouble, then getting out of trouble, and then laying low for a while, and then off I would go again through the same loop.

I was a binge drinker. I could go for long periods without incident and then I would take off on a bender. Later on in my drinking career I would hole up in a hotel for a week until I could stop. I had a conviction for driving under the influence in 1980, some nine years before I came into AA. I was forced to go to therapy and classes—but I manipulated and lied my way through them because I knew it was safe to do that, and that I wasn't ready to stop yet. I really believed at the time that I didn't have a problem.

I reached a point late in 1989 where I just knew I couldn't continue the way I had been and that something had to change. I was sick of the person I saw in the mirror, and, emotionally, I was at the bottom.

I asked for help and I was given it.

The Importance of Hitting Bottom

The addiction cycle can be broken, and successful management calls for combining physiological, psychological, socio-cultural and biological factors but none of these will be effective if the addict does not want to stop. Success can occur only when the alcoholic can see the true nature of his/her malady and has a willingness to go to any length to treat it. AA founder Bill Wilson viewed the active alcoholic as "an extreme example of self-will run riot." And he believed that a complete desperation or a devastating humbling, known as "hitting bottom" was absolutely necessary to driving the alcoholic to embrace the willingness to do whatever it will take to stay sober. As Wilson wrote in Twelve Steps and Twelve Traditions:

> Only through utter defeat are we able to take the first steps towards liberation and strength … Our admission of personal powerlessness finally turns out to be the firm bedrock upon which happy and purposeful lives may be built.[93]

It is on this premise that the Twelve Steps of Alcoholics Anonymous are built. It is only when the alcoholic abstains from alcohol, and thereby arrests the allergy, that the other aspects of the disease can be treated.

In the following case study, Rick was not able to stop drinking when his loving family tried to help or even when he was admitted to a detox unit. It was not until he surrendered his will and his alcoholism to a higher power in a simple prayer that the torturous obsession was lifted from him. He was able to stop drinking when the truth of his disease could no longer be denied within himself. Hitting bottom is the admission of defeat that you alone cannot stop drinking, and that without help you will most surely die. This is the first step of the twelve steps of Alcoholics Anonymous: "We admitted we were powerless over alcohol and that our lives had become unmanageable." [94]

Case Study:
Rick W's Story

"Alcohol Called the Shots"

I am Rick W., one of eight children born to Dan and Patricia. I was born the second son, after my brother Dan, who is two years older than I am. I was never the student my older brother was, nor did I have his looks, wit, athletic ability, or other attributes. In many ways, I may have been jealous. My younger siblings are Julie, then Christopher, David, Maribeth, Jane and the youngest, Stephen. We were the typical large Catholic family, and we all got along with each other. We went to Parochial school in Melrose, Massachusetts. I consider myself blessed to have had the parents I do. They shared equally in the huge responsibility of raising eight kids.

My childhood memories are, for the most part, really wonderful. Our home was warm and loving, and I had a constant sense of security. Like most kids, I often wondered what it would be like to live in the homes of some of my friends who didn't have the same rules and discipline that we had to follow at our house.

One of my earliest traumas was when I was singled out in first grade for having an accident. I wet myself and the nun put my chair on a desk and I had to sit there. This taught me to avoid that kind of humiliation at any cost. I became terrified of being singled out or laughed at. This kept me from participating in many activities.

Academically, I did all right with applied effort—which I didn't always put forth. But applying myself did not matter that much after I got drunk for the first time—on wine in the seventh grade. Suddenly, I was the center of attention with my friends. I acted foolishly, crashed my bike, threw up, and couldn't wait to do it again! Although I couldn't get booze very easily at age eleven, I became obsessed with it. After that first episode, it, the booze, started calling the shots in my life, and it dictated the direction that I would follow.

Slowly my values began to change. Things I would never have thought of doing at one time suddenly became "not so bad". Bending and breaking the rules became more routine. I started seeking out new friends, gravitating toward kids in public school, or those who were from single parent homes that had more lenient rules to follow. I can see now that the instant gratification and the quick fix was what I wanted. This was to be the ground work for about 23 years of progressive alcoholism.

My disease took me from myself from the early stages and kept taking until the time I surrendered to it. Experiences with family, friendships, education, anything that came between me and booze got shoved aside. Needless to say, this didn't go unnoticed by those closest to me. Help was offered at the earliest sign there was a problem—by my parents trying to direct me away from certain friends. As the trouble increased, more drastic offers appeared, i.e.: AA!

Back in those days, AA was very much more hush-hush than it is today. I did, however, know of one friend's father who used to be the neighborhood drunk and after attending AA meetings had changed noticeably.

Fast forward fifteen years. I have lost jobs, relationships, trust, careers, everything. I went to three or four detox's, but I was trying to stop for all the wrong reasons. All of these things, along with court ordered attendance at AA meetings, helped me find my way into recovery. Booze, however, was the final convincer.

One time after I had been asked to leave a detox, I bought a fifth of vodka and drank most of it on the cab ride to the apartment at which I was staying. It was there I realized the alcohol wasn't doing what it had always done in the past. I was drunk from the neck down. I couldn't stop my head from realizing I was devastated! I fell on the bed and cried out a prayer from deep inside asking God to please help me … He did.

I thought to call someone who had given me their phone number. That led to other calls to central service and other AA's who responded in true AA fashion. I was being taken care of. That was December 15, 1982. I started attendance at meetings and doing all that was suggested except paying attention to what they said regarding substitutes! I used recreational drugs off and on for another year or so.

On April 10th, 1984, my sobriety date, I was released from the obsession to take any mood or mind altering substances. That was the day before I started an AWOLL program where I was told we had to get really honest about everything. Thank God! Recovery has been a wonderful journey. I joined a group, the "4 Winds" in Malden, Massachusetts, and got a sponsor. I collected lots of phone numbers and I learned to use them. I got active in AA. I've had all the jobs there are in A.A.: I go on commitments, twelfth step calls, and try to carry the message in everyday life—in and out of the AA program.

Every area of my life has improved as a result of getting sober. I have a relationship with the God of my understanding that continues to broaden and deepen and increase my faith in Him. This spiritual healing and wellness overflows into the other areas of my thoughts, feelings, life.

The obsession was lifted—taken away—and that's a freedom beyond description for an alcoholic/addict. Realizing how sobriety has illuminated the precious gift of life, I want to improve the quality of my life all the time. I try to read spiritual material and information pertaining to recovery. I am completely grateful to God for bringing my wife into my life. With our children, friends, and family always close, I think: "How could there not be a God who only wants to love us all the time no matter what?" I am so blessed.

My life today stays centered on recovery first. I attend three to four meetings per week. I attend Mass with my family most Sundays. My wife and I practice meditation daily, and pray together whenever possible. Exercise is also a constant in my life, with sports, golf, skiing, biking, camping, and just about anything outdoors. I attend two to three AA retreats each year, one for couples, and two for men in recovery.

The three key elements for me would be: meetings; sponsorship; and seeing God do for me time and time again what I could never do for myself.

I wish love and good luck to anyone seeking such a path.

The first step is said to be the only step a recovering alcoholic has to do perfectly. Accepting powerlessness is an absolute, so the abstinence from alcohol must be absolute as well. The foundation of the program of alcoholics anonymous is based on arresting the physical aspect of the disease by total abstinence because when an alcoholic drinks he/she cannot predict the outcome. Accepting this fact is the beginning of recovery.

The Nutritional Damage of Alcoholism

All alcoholics are malnourished to a certain extent, because alcohol consumption affects the body's ability to absorb nutrients. Abstinence alone cannot reverse structural damage done at the cellular level. Vitamins, minerals, amino acids, and such are all needed in therapeutic amounts over lengthy periods of time so that the body can begin to heal itself.

Hypoglycemia, or chronic low blood sugar, is often found in second- and third-stage alcoholics due to the compromised functions in the liver and endocrine system. Hypoglycemic symptoms include: headache, fatigue, anxiety, depression, fuzzy thinking, shakiness, weakness, irritability, sleeplessness, hunger, and forgetfulness. These symptoms can appear to be psychological, but should not be assumed to be such until the alcoholic's diet is carefully studied. Following a hypoglycemic diet—one based on frequent small meals throughout the day and the elimination of refined carbohydrates such as found in "junk food" and sweets—can be an important tool in preventing relapse. Another important factor in alleviating depression and extreme fatigue can be Vitamin B therapy. Heavy drinking can limit the body's ability to absorb thiamine (B1) and Pyridoxine (B-6). [95] Zinc, Calcium, magnesium, potassium, and phosphorus are minerals essential to feeling well and energized. Zinc plays an especially important role in metabolizing alcohol in the liver, and its elimination from the body due to protracted heavy drinking over time precludes normal liver function. [96]

Depression has been linked in some cases to calcium loss, and studies have shown marked improvement in some patients taking this and other supplements. The treatment includes supplementing tryptophan, calcium, magnesium, and niacin. Tryptophan is essential to the formation of serotonin, a neurotransmitter in the brain that helps to control moods.[97] A glucose tolerance test will show if a recovering alcoholic is suffering from hypoglycemia and depression due to mineral deficiencies. Dr. August F. Daro, a Chicago obstetrician, states, "Low blood sugar is the most common cause of depression, though it is not commonly diagnosed." He recommends a diet rich in protein and free of sugars, coffee and refined carbohydrates.

Glutamine in Treatment of Alcoholism

In the 1950's, important research was conducted at the University of Oklahoma by Dr. R.J. Williams using nutritional supplements to control the intake of alcohol by alcoholics. In this ten-year study, the amino acid, L-glutamine, was given to ten subjects who each had been drinking heavily over a period of three months. There appeared to be a marked improvement in each subject's ability to stay away from a drink.[98] More research is needed, but the results were very promising in showing that glutamine may be an important supplement in the control and recovery phases of alcoholism.[99]

Dr. Jose Ordovas, director of the Nutrition and Genomics Laboratory at Tuffs University believes, "It isn't just what you eat that can kill you, and it isn't just your DNA that can save you—it's how they interact."[100] Ordovas says, "Within a decade, doctors will be able to take genetic profiles of their patients, identify specific diseases for which they are at risk, and create customized nutrition plans."[101] Based on the current knowledge of how nutritional deficiencies affect the alcoholic and the recovering alcoholic, this is very exciting news that may lead to more effective treatment.

Treating the Psychological Disease of Alcoholism

The effectiveness of treatment in counseling an alcoholic has a crucial dependence on his/her acceptance of the reality that he/she is powerless over alcohol and that nothing short of total abstinence will arrest the disease. This principle is the cornerstone of Alcoholics Anonymous. The next step is to recognize that alcoholism is also mental illness. Step two, in the Twelve Step program states: "… came to believe that a power greater than ourselves could restore us to sanity". Sanity means wholeness, and the concept of this second step can be summed up in the Latin phrase: Mens sana in corpore sano, which roughly translates, sane mind in a sane body. The insane behavior of an active alcoholic is not alcoholism but it is the byproduct of alcoholism. It is believed by many professionals that alcoholism is a symptom of an underlying disorder, and while that may be true, it does not change the physical allergy to alcohol. The argument as to whether an alcoholic drinks because of his/her emotional illness or becomes emotionally ill as a result of his/her drinking is irrelevant.

Alcoholism is a three-fold disease, body, mind, and spirit, and all three dimensions need individualized treatment based on the patient's specific needs.

The mind and the emotions of a recovering alcoholic are often confused, and it takes time to sort out truth from delusion. Proper diet can help a great deal in speeding up this process. For many recovering alcoholics the program of AA with its sponsorship and fellowship support is enough for them to achieve long-lasting sober thinking and, consequently, mental sobriety. There are those alcoholics that have a more complex emotional make-up or two separate, completely different disorders, which need to be treated by professionals. In seeking a professional, whether a psychotherapist, psychologist, psychiatrist, or medical doctor, it is critical to ask if that professional has training in the field of alcoholism and is aware of the tenets of Alcoholics Anonymous. Treatment should not be confused with recovery.

> Treatment is a linear approach, connoting an intense set of actions for a limited period of time—treatment, aftercare and follow-up. Recovery, on the other hand, is a way of life with no categories or degrees—just newcomers and old-timers.[102]

Treating the Spiritual Disease of Alcoholism

William Miller, director of the University of New Mexico's Center for Research on Addictive Behaviors writes:

> I am puzzling over the fact that broad, dramatic and persistent changes, which might properly be called transformations or conversions, do occur in human lives, and seem to be much more common outside of formal treatment ... These transformations are considered normal in AA.[103]

Researchers and treatment professionals often have difficulty understanding the spiritual aspect of the disease of alcoholism. Of great help in bridging the gap between psychology and spirituality was the approach of Carl Jung. In January of 1961, Jung wrote in a letter to Bill Wilson, "Alcohol in Latin is spiritis, and you use the same word for the highest religious experience as well as for the most depraving poison. The helpful formula therefore is: Spiritus contra spiritum." Jung understood as few had before the spiritual sickness the alcoholic experiences. He knew that unless the alcoholic had a conversion experience or as we call it today, a spiritual awakening, long term sobriety is more than likely impossible.

Miller speaks of this conflict in the approach to the disease, "We research expectancies; self-image; defense mechanism; DNA; enzymes; neurochemicals; immune function; and the influence of gender, culture, and advertising. But the spiritual dimension is curiously ignored."[104]

Transpersonal psychology (body, mind, and spirit psychology) in the treatment of the alcoholic and the alcoholic's family has had tremendous success. Virtually every leader in the field of addiction today has incorporated transpersonal psychology in their work. Robert DuPont, former NIDA chief who heads both the Institute for Behavioral Health, and a consulting firm in the Washington, D.C. area has been very instrumental in bringing the understanding of spiritual health to the treatment field, noting, "We in the scientific community have to accept that the spiritual component is the key to getting well." He goes on to explain, "The scientific people think it's religious and not scientific. It's not religious and it is scientific. Spirituality is very simply the antidote to self-centeredness that is the core of addiction and mental illness."[105]

Working with others is an important part of the AA fellowship. A common phrase is, "Give it away to keep it." AA members never graduate and never stop working on their conscious contact with a power greater than themselves:

> I sought my soul, and it escaped me.
> I sought my God, and He eluded me.
> I sought my brother, and I found all three.
>
>   Anonymous

7

ALCOHOLISM: TREATABLE, NOT CURABLE

The issue of health care reform cannot be adequately addressed until we decide to deal with the problem of addiction.

—Joseph Califano,
Former U.S. Secretary of
Health, Education & Welfare

Alcoholism and drug addiction cost the nation approximately $300 billion per year.[106] This staggering cost in health and productivity makes addiction one of the most costly and serious problems facing our nation today. These costs continue to rise annually, and the need for more effective and efficient treatment models is obvious. Society spends ten times as much on social-related costs due to active alcoholism than it does on treatment for the disease.[107] What is the most effective treatment for alcoholism? It is now well known that genetic, as well as, psychological, environmental, and social factors contribute to addiction. This is why no treatment that focuses on only one aspect of the disease will be effective in the long run. Adding to the problem is the on-going controversy surrounding alcoholism treatment. Currently, the most widespread and effective treatment is rooted in the 12 steps of Alcoholics Anonymous but science is exploring the use of drugs, such as naltrexone, that block the brain's receptors for opioids. This mimics the feeling of euphoria often associated with drinking alcohol.[108] Exploring the idea that if you can "fool" the pleasure centers of the brain through such medications will the desire to drink alcohol be removed?

According to Llyoyd Vacovsky, Executive Director, American Council on Alcoholism, there are currently three mainstream treatment approaches for chemical dependency; the Minnesota Model (based on the 12 step program of Alcoholics Anonymous and the Hazelden Treatment Center program), cognitive behavioral psychotherapy, and pharmacotherapy (the Pennsylvania Model, a medical model based on the research at the Pennsylvania School of Medicine).

The Minnesota Model

The Hazelden Treament Center began in 1949 as a guest house for male alcoholics. Alcoholics and their families faced very dim prospects for recovery before that time. Alcoholics Anonymous (founded in 1935) was still new and relatively unknown in most parts of the country, so the desperate alcoholic was either shipped off to a mental ward at a private or state hospital (in the early days known as the "snake pit"), arrested and sent to prison or died prematurely as a result of alcohol related illness. The skid row bum which is the image often associated with alcoholics is often in reality the third stage alcoholic waiting to die. Even though society still can witness alcoholics at the margins of existence on the streets of their communities, there are many other options open to alcoholics and drug addicts if they choose to utilize them. These treatment options are due in part to the extraordinary efforts of the early pioneers of A.A. and Hazelden. This former guest house for alcoholic men has become the foremost method for treating alcoholics in this country and abroad. Famous facilities like the Betty Ford Center, which share the same multidisciplinary approach to treatment, often combine forces for fundraising and research projects with Hazelden.

Gordon Grimm, a former Lutheran minister, was one of the pioneers of the Minnesota Model. From 1966 to 1970 under the guidance of Grimm, the multidisciplinary approach to alcoholism treatment was to take shape and become known as the Minnesota Model. Robert M. Morse, MD, director of the Mayo Clinic in Rochester, Minnesota explains, "Historically, it represents a very important step forward in its insistence on alcoholism as a primary disease. The model flourished in the absence of real alternatives. It remains a treatment model most predictive of success." The model was the first humane approach to the treatment of alcoholism. It is "holistic" in nature, and although it incorporates the practice and fellowship of Alcoholics Anonymous in its treatment plan it also utilizes Jungian psychology, Albert Ellis' Rational—Emotive Therapy, (RET) Skinner's peer group therapy, A.A. meetings, and more. It is also committed to addressing all the problems that may face the recovering addict, including depression, attention deficit, and various forms of adult and childhood abuse and so on.[109] Gordon Grimm who retired after 30 years of service to Hazelden in 1995 states, "I like to view the work of Hazelden as a continually evolving process of caring for people—one that has been modeled worldwide, one that has helped change and improve the way society deals with alcoholics."

Defining the Minnesota Model and explaining how if differs from other addiction treatments is best left to one of the key developers of the model and the president emeritus of Hazelden Foundation, Daniel J. Anderson, PhD. Anderson describes the model as a set of "core perspectives:

- Treat the alcoholic with respect. Alcoholics are sick people, not bad people.

- Treat alcoholism as a chronic illness—one that calls for coping not curing, understanding not shaming.

- Treat alcoholics and addicts "holistically". The illness affects people in many different ways. Treatment should involve physical, spiritual, psychological, and social areas.

- Treatment should offer diagnosis, detoxification, aftercare, Twelve Step attendance, and family therapy.

- Offer to the recovering alcoholic the expertise of medicine, psychotherapy, spirituality/religion, nutrition etc.

- Stress the importance of lifelong abstinence and the commitment to the fellowship and the principals of Alcoholics Anonymous.

- Peer counseling and camaraderie as important tools for maintaining sobriety.[110]

Author Jerry Spicer writes in his book, The Minnesota Model: The Evolutionary Approach to Addiction Recovery:

> The Minnesota Model represents a social reform movement that humanizes the treatment of people addicted to alcohol and other drugs … we cannot assume that this movement is complete. The "war on drugs" too easily becomes the war on people who take drugs.[111]

A perfect example of the caring and respect that the counselors and staff at Hazelden give to their patients is illustrated in Bob's story. In this case study, Bob is admitted to the Hazelden program but he has a slip after 25 days of sobriety. The foundation of treatment he received there planted seeds of recovery that would eventually save his life:

Case Study:
Bob's Story

"One Drink Was All It Took"

I was born and raised in a lower middle class family, and can't recall any alcoholism in my family. My father, on occasion, would drive me to the local bar on Sundays. I would sit in a booth and play some of the electronic games, drink cokes and eat snacks while he watched football and had a few beers with the boys. But I don't believe he was an alcoholic. What I do remember vividly is one time when I was about 5 years old I took a sip of his beer and it was like electricity running through me and I knew that I would have that again. And so the journey had begun.

At 12 years old, I officially began my consistent drinking and drugging career. For years I enjoyed the pleasures and good feelings that the chemicals brought me. They were short-lived, and the good times began to change to desperate ones in my early to middle 20's. I found myself drinking and taking drugs on a daily basis.

By society's standards, I appeared to be a success. At 19 I started my business—which I still have today—and purchased my first house—with many more to follow. However, as I look back I always felt empty and unfulfilled. Nothing seemed to have any value.

As time went on, my alcoholism accelerated quickly to the point where I ended up living in the attic of one of my apartment houses, strung out on heroin and lying in bed with a quart of vodka next to me. I traded anything I could for a drink and a bag of heroin, and became the type of person that I loathed. My parents taught me the values that create good moral fiber, including ethics, honesty, kindness, etc., but I traded each and every one of them just for a fix. I lived and believed in all those values at one time and came to the point where I lived by none of them. I hated myself and what I had become. When it finally sunk in that I was too deep and couldn't stop on my own, I became riddled with fear that I was hopeless and I would die before I reach 30 years of age.

I sought out a psychiatrist who was also in Alcoholics Anonymous, and he told me that I had a disease and that I needed a divine intervention if I was to recover. He sent me to Hazelden Rehabilitation Center in Minnesota. I was clean for 25 days, but I knew deep inside that I wasn't done with drinking and drugging. I bought some pills and drank while I was there. I came down from that high with help of the counselors there and then I got kicked out. I flew home. My first day back I bought a case of beer and a quart of vodka and 3 bags of heroin. I did go to AA meetings for about a week or two even while I was drinking. I eventually stopped and stayed actively drinking until May 5,

1982 which I pray to God was and always will be my last drinking and drug taking experience.

On that day, I was in the middle of drinking and using heroin. I was so depressed that I was suicidal. However, instead of continuing with that intent, I got down on my knees and begged God to help me. That was the divine intervention that my psychiatrist was talking about because my obsession and compulsion to continue to use drugs and alcohol completely stopped and I was lifted on the spot. Instead of going to the bar, I went home, took a shower, got dressed, and just sat on my couch for hours waiting for an AA meeting to start. That was May 5, 1982.

I would say that fear and desperation were assets to me in early sobriety. I was told to get a sponsor, and I did that immediately. Together, we dove into the 12 steps of recovery. I attended no fewer than two meetings per day, and I completed the suggested 90/90 (90 meetings in 90 days). I have been very consistent in attending 5–7 AA meetings per week. The longer I stay sober, the more I realize what a gift and blessing I have been freely given. The backbone of my life is provided by God (a higher power) and by Alcoholics Anonymous.

I believe the 12 steps of recovery are an absolute must for me and for anyone who wants to stay in recovery. I firmly believe that straying from AA, perhaps believing that 22 years of sobriety enable me to go it alone, would be insanity, and bring the certain failure of drink and/or drugs.

The benefits of sobriety are limitless, but I can think of a few right now. I have become, and continue to strive to be the man that I want to be and one of whom I believe God approves. I can't say that I have always been happy and free of myself in sobriety, but I do feel consistently free and happy now. Several years ago, I started to spend more time in meditation and prayer to my God. Each day, I ask Him for guidance, and also for a person to come into my life each day who can use my help. Through his kindness and love for me, He has fulfilled this request each day. It is clear to me now that the more I give, the better I feel about myself. I've had many difficulties developing a faith and a trust in my God, but now my belief is strong. My spirits are basically high and when He puts someone into my life that I can help, I thank him for the opportunity. I believe that the more I focus on the 11th step—prayer—the more spiritual awakenings I have, and the more my life improves. I have a responsibility to give away what was and is still freely given to me. My message to anyone in AA is to never quit, especially when going through a difficult life situation. "Time and effort" has brought me to some wonderful places I would never have experienced if I were drinking. I love being sober and an active member of Alcoholics Anonymous, and feel it is a gift that I need to protect and nurture.

I believe some of the key elements to my 22+ years of sobriety have been consistency and a craving for growth in sobriety. The three-fold disease of alcoholism is alive and well within me, and keeps me aware that I need to stay very close to AA, to my discipline with physical exercise, and to my attentiveness to God. When I first sobered up, I was very active with exercise, and have stayed consistent with it, working out at least 5 or 6 days per week, by way of cardiovascular exercise, free weights, or yoga. I also know that the more time I spend with prayer and meditation, or simply in talking to my God as I would talk to you, the greater my sense of inner peace. I have gone from a belief in God to a faith in God, and now to a trust in God.

I'm a big fan of the AA steps "don't drink" and "Go to meetings." I am aware that there is more to sobriety, but if I'm not drinking and am attending as many meetings as possible, I hear and learn the things that are necessary to a fulfilling and contented life.

The Minnesota Model believes that alcoholism is a disease that is spiritual in nature, and that by re-establishing spiritual values through developing a relationship with a Higher Power, long term recovery is possible. In Bob's story he tells us that he has gone from "a belief in God to a faith in God" and that this is a key element in his long term sobriety. The other crucial element is being an active member of A.A.

Treatment for alcoholism alone will not keep an alcoholic sober, a belief in a Higher Power alone will not keep an alcoholic sober, someone's love and devotion alone will not keep an alcoholic sober (as many a member of Al-Anon will attest), attending A.A. meetings alone will not keep an alcoholic sober. None of these things alone can guarantee sobriety. It is only when the alcoholic hits a personal and internal "bottom" and the truth of his/her malady is revealed that a complete surrender is possible. It is only when the addict is willing to go to any lengths to stay sober that all of the above actions become life-saving tools capable of transforming the addict's life.

Intervention

Intervention involves family and friends confronting the active alcoholic about his/her alcoholism, and the effect it has had on their lives. It is facilitated by a professional with very specific guidelines. The ultimate goal is to have the alcoholic acknowledge his/her drinking problem and become willing, regardless of how reluctant he/she is to get treatment. Before confronting the alcoholic, the family and friends are taken through a process with a professional which involves: educating them on the disease of alcoholism, treatment options for the alcoholic and the family system; devising a treatment plan if the alcoholic is willing to get help, understanding "enabling" behaviors and learning the principals that help everyone out of denial and into a fair assessment of the current situation; and collecting stories and incidents to share with the alcoholic about their behavior and how it has effected each person participating. Finally, after the family and friends are clear and a rehearsal has been completed, a confrontation with the alcoholic takes place. The intervention process is an important tool and can be very successful in many cases if executed correctly and with love and caring. Former First Lady, Betty Ford recalls in an interview how her family's intervention saved her life and got her on the road to recovery:

> My daughter, Susan, and my gynecologist tried to do a small intervention. I practically threw them out of the house. Fortunately, they were not deterred—they went back and got the troops. The second intervention involved the whole family plus two physicians. It was hard for me to buck. First, I was very glad to see all my family, delighted they were paying so much attention to me. When I realized they were addressing the fact that I had a problem with alcohol and drugs, I became very angry. Finally, I began to painfully realize that I had failed as a wife and a mother of this family. Yet I kept hearing them say they loved me too much to let me go. And I began to see the sunlight.[112]

Betty Ford, through her commitment to her own sobriety and the sobriety of others, went on to establish the Betty Ford Center in Rancho Mirage, California. The Betty Ford Center also collaborates with other treatment centers such as Hazelden to help deliver quality, cost-effective care to alcoholics and their families by using the basics of the Minnesota Model. Mrs. Ford explains, "We have both interventionists and family treatment. We believe in a holistic approach to treatment—offering everything from nutrition to physical activity to spiritual renewal." (p. 29)

Cognitive Behavioral Therapy

The second approach, according to Lloyd Vacovsky, Executive Director of the American Council on Alcoholism, and principal in the treatment group, Assisted Recovery Centers of America (ARCA), believes that treatment should be drawn according to individual needs. Each case should be evaluated with an awareness of the biological and behavioral aspects of the disease in that individual. Some individual cases will call for pharmacological treatment. The treatment approach uses therapeutic techniques to evaluate the damage done from the abuse of alcohol and how to make changes to amend this destructive behavior to make better choices in the future. This technique uses one-on-one counseling, rather than group counseling. It also includes evaluating and constructing a treatment plan that encompasses the individual's biological, environmental, psychological, and psycho-spiritual condition. More information on cognitive behavioral therapy can be found on Vacovsky's website: www.assistedrecovery.com.

The Albert Ellis Institute in New York City was founded in 1968 and is considered the founder of Rational Emotive Behavioral Therapy (REBT), an action-based program for personal growth and empowerment addressing the psychological and social issues of the addict in a supportive therapeutic setting. Behavioral techniques may work for a problem drinker but will not necessarily work for an alcoholic whose disease is extremely complex and still progressing. Alcoholism, being a three-fold disease—physical, mental, and spiritual, must be treated as such.

In light of the latest brain research suggesting that the brain is the site of alcoholism, neuroscientists must continue to study the various neurotransmitters and receptor subtypes involved in the development of alcoholism. This is why the Pennsylvania model is so interesting, involving as it does both cognitive behavioral counseling and a strong medical and scientific research component to evaluate and develop proper treatment of the individual.

The Pennsylvania Model

This model is based on clinical studies and research conducted by the University of Pennsylvania in the last 20 years. It represents a medical model that expands treatment to include pharmacotherapy. Pharmacotherapy combines cognitive behavioral therapy with the use medications that address the biological components of the disease of alcoholism.[113]

Medication developed for the treatment of alcoholism has three main goals: treatment of the withdrawal symptoms, deterrents, and maintenance of abstinence. The psychopharmacological revolution began in the 1950's with the discovery of medications that could subdue the mentally ill. Since 1955, many new chemical agents have been developed to treat many disorders in the field of mental illness such as phenothiazines and benzodiazepines.[114] Benzodiazepines (Valium for example) are currently used to treat withdrawal symptoms in alcoholics and addicts because they stop the racing sympathetic nervous system which can cause seizures.[115] For many years there was a refusal in the medical community to medicate alcoholics and addicts through the withdrawal phase. Old prejudices and attitudes prevailed, based on the belief that "If they don't suffer they

will just get cleaned up and go back out there again." Fortunately, those old attitudes have faded and effective, humane treatment is available thanks to these
drugs and caring professionals. In the 1990s Anatabuse (disulfiram) was introduced to serve as a deterrent. The person taking the medication will often experience severe and unpleasant symptoms if he/she drinks alcohol. It is used as part of
treatment plan but it is by no means a solution to alcohol abuse.[116]

According to a February, 2005 news release by Health Behavior News Service,
the University of Pennsylvania has been conducting research on the drug naltrexone (marketed as ReVia) for relapse prevention since the 1980's.[117] (Kennedy,
2005, para 6). The drug has been proven effective in reducing the risk of relaps-
ing into heavy drinking within the first three months of recovery by 36% and also
in lowering by 18% the chances of a patient in treatment quitting his/her program.[118] Naltrexone does not prevent a person from drinking, but it can have a
positive effect on the amount that a person drinks. Dr. Joseph Volpicelli and the
U.S. Substance Abuse and Mental Health Services Administration agree that
abstinence is the only effective method for arresting alcoholism but Volpicelli
argues, "20 million Americans suffer from alcohol abuse disorders, yet only about
2 million are in any kind of treatment program. We should be flexible enough to
get at the 90% who are not in treatment."[119] I feel strongly that the current
trend of scientific research will prove to have a tremendous effect on the identification, treatment, and stabilization of the disease of alcoholism in the next
decade. It is my hope that the tide is turning on this epidemic and that we may all
one day see a primarily sober society where alcoholism is diagnosed and treated at
the level that it exists and that no alcoholic falls through the cracks of denial
again.

Dr. Volpicelli believes that craving is an important component in reinforcing
the use and abuse of alcohol as well as a major factor in relapse. He points out
that because "craving is a neuro-chemical reaction, it is best treated with medications." [120]

The field of addiction and treatment is evolving rapidly as research into the
inner workings of the brain continues. The understanding among treatment professionals that alcoholism and many forms of addiction are diseases of the brain is
slowly being acknowledged. Research by the NIDA and the NIAAA has produced startling evidence on how alcohol abuse can lead the user across "an invisible biobehavioral line". [121] Once this line is crossed, as visualized through the
use of brain-imaging technology, doctors can witness the alterations in the alco-
holic/addict's brain. This technology has changed the diagnosis of alcoholism
from being a metaphorical disease to a "true biobehavioral disease".[122] Perhaps

the definition will expand even more to include both diagnoses'. The metaphorical or spiritual aspect of the disease, which has been so effectively treated with the 12 steps of Alcoholics Anonymous, and psychotherapy can join forces with the newly emerging field of brain research to administer effective medications, when necessary, on the currently untreated U.S. population of alcoholics, estimated at about 20 million people. The improvements to be gained by individuals in the quality of their lives and those of their family members, in addition to added effectiveness of the billions spent each year on healthcare and social programs would be extraordinary.

Exploring Other Treatment Models

At the Life management Center in Minneapolis founder and author, Bernie Larsen teaches family therapy groups. As a former Catholic priest he offers valuable skills to people wanting to recover from the effects of being raised in an alcoholic home and/or their own alcoholism. He teaches five essential skills for recovery:

- The ability to take personal responsibility. Blaming others has to stop if we are to gain self-esteem. Saying "no" to any abuse in any form, no matter what.

- The ability to ask for what you need and/or to say how you feel.

- The ability to fight fair. To resist the temptation to go for the jugular-you may win the fight, but loose the war.

- The ability to create and maintain a safe living environment for yourself and your family.

- The ability to only use positive emotional tools for solving one's problems.[123]

The issue of personal responsibility is again reinforced in Dr. David Smith's and Richard Seymour's book, *Drugfree: A Unique, Positive Approach to Staying Off Alcohol and Other Drugs*. Dr. Smith observes, "They may not be responsible for their addictions, but they are definitely responsible for their recovery."[124] Their book outlines a blueprint for recovery which includes hypnosis, yoga, meditation, acupuncture, lucid dreaming, nutrition and massage. They believe that these practices can provide long term healing and spiritual growth.

Glide Church in San Francisco has developed a very unique recovery approach for African-Americans under the tutelage of Reverend Cecil Williams. In the late 1960's he opened the doors to his church to help the sick and suffering addicts at the height of the drug revolution. He observed that even though the 12 steps of Alcoholics Anonymous had tremendous success, some of its practices were not as helpful to the African-American population. "African-Americans are communal people; we fight for freedom together ... A black person hears the call to powerlessness as one more command to lie down and take it."[125] He developed four "acts" on the way to recovery:

• Recognition—uncovering the secrets, the behaviors and the feelings surrounding our addictions.

• Self-Definition—Find out who you are and stand tall in that truth.

• Rebirth—The public declaration of who we are from the inside out.

• Community—Develop relations with all our brothers and sisters of all colors and classes. (pp 42–44)

Perhaps one of the most unique and controversial approaches to the treatment of addiction is the Lenair Technique. It was brought to the United States by Dr. Winston Marlowe. It was adopted by Rhonda Lenair, who at 16 years old in the early 1970's suddenly fell ill during an audition for the London Ballet Festival. She was diagnosed with a mass in her abdomen, for which surgery was recommended. During this time, she met with Dr. Winston Marlowe, who had studied healing treatments using electromagnetic and bioelectric energy fields in the former Soviet Union and Poland. Lenair became interested in Marlowe's non-surgical healing methodologies and decided to forego the recommended surgery. The mass disappeared on its own after a short time. She became Dr. Marlowe's protégé, and over the next decade further developed the electromagnetic techniques to which Dr. Marlowe had introduced her, establishing a practice in Boston in 1987 based on their use. Her electromagnetic procedures are recognized for their effectiveness in helping people quickly end addictions.[126] According to a 1989 follow-up survey of 500 patients, 92% were successfully treated.[127] Many of her clients are employed as healthcare professionals, including the well-known author Dr. Christine Northrup, who espouses the health benefits of the technique and personally recommends it.

In light of this new technology and medical research, one can assume that the developments in the field of addiction in the next decade are expected to be very exciting and its impact on society as a whole far reaching to say the least. It is here that perhaps treatment professionals can take a word of advice from the program of Alcoholics Anonymous when it suggests to its members to employ the slogan H.O.W. it works: Honesty, Open-Mindedness and Willingness.

> If we can honestly look at the new medications and treatments and keep an open mind about the scientific research, and are willing to expand our own knowledge of how best to treat an individual patient, perhaps we can finally bring this chronic epidemic under a healthy system of control, and not pass it on to another generation.

8

INSIDE ALCOHOLICS ANONYMOUS

Alcoholics Anonymous

Alcoholics Anonymous is an integral part of the Hazelden treatment program which is also identified as a spiritual program. A.A. refers to itself not as a treatment program but rather a fellowship of individuals with the common desire to not drink, one day at a time. The Twelve Steps are the tools by which the alcoholic can achieve that goal. According to the American Medical Association, "... treatment primarily involves not taking a drink ..." Anyone who has been in the grips of active alcoholism or has known a loved one with the disease knows that this is no easy feat. "Alcoholics Anonymous is the most successful lay movement for alcoholics in the last 200 years." remarks A.A. historian and consultant, Bill Pittman. So how does A.A. help the recovering alcoholic heal the physical, psychological and spiritual damage brought about by active addiction so that lifelong sobriety may be achieved? A.A. has three important components; the 12 steps (which is the program of recovery), sponsorship (which serves as a lay therapist and/or mentor for working the program) and the fellowship (which is the group of like minded individuals sharing a common disease and commitment to stay sober one day at a time and to go to any length to achieve that goal by supporting one another.

In Matt's case history, a 30-day treatment facility gave him the opportunity to experience sobriety for the first time since he was 12 years old. It was exhilarating, but he soon discovered that he would not be able to maintain it without the program of A.A. and the support of a caring sponsor:

Case Study:
Matt's Story

"Rehab or Jail"—That Was the Choice"

My first drink was at age of twelve in 1966 at a Jamestown annual picnic called Family Day. I drank a bottle of scotch, ending up extremely sick and falling off a tractor into bees nest. I was stung over 50 times, and made a scene in front of whole town, disgracing my family. Consequently, I was grounded for over a year.

My father was soon to take an assignment at the Pentagon. A Navy Captain, he was appointed by the Joint Chiefs of Staff in 1967, when the family moved with him to Washington, in the midst of the race riots in Washington DC and other American cities. I remember sneaking out of house and joining friends to drink grain alcohol and watch the fires burning in Washington. Around that time I also started to experiment with hashish given to me by one of my brothers, but I ratted on him, for which he never forgave me.

An eighth grade teacher tried to molest me, and I'll never forget the guilt. He lost his job. I moved to Rochester NY for my high school years, as between 1969 and 1973 my father was stationed at the University of Rochester, where he headed the ROTC program. I was highly dyslexic and was having a hard time sitting still in class. Reading and writing were very difficult, but I was very athletic, and because I was extremely outgoing, had a lot of friends. I was the life of the party!!!

I attended Catholic high school and felt I had been very sexually repressed. I fell in love with a girl from Ireland named Mary—the same name as my mother. She overwhelmed my life, but drinking soon took over instead. Drinking made me feel great inside … until the next day. I had blackouts and used to do wild things to impress my friends. We streaked through the brothers' quarters and into the nun's quarters and, of course, got caught and were ordered to wash police cars for one year.

At the age of 16 I had my first drunk-driving accident. I went through a stop sign with my prized first vehicle: a red pick up truck, slamming into the side of a brand new car driven by a 17 year old girl. Her mother came into the police station and tried to attack me, and the cops almost arrested her—and let me go.

My senior year, Mary, my love, told me to hit the highway because of my drinking and newfound friend, marijuana. I made it through high school, although I'm not sure how, and was accepted at Paul Smith College of Forestry in the Adirondack Mountains in New York near Saranac Lake, a town with more bars per capita than any town in the Nation. The bars are open until four in the morning, and alcoholism runs rampant. My nickname was 'Bong', after a marijuana smoking pipe very popular at the time. I got into bar room fights, had sex with local girls without protection, and suffered worsening guilt about it all. In my schoolwork, I cheated as much as much as possible to get by—and thought I was living the good life!

With the forestry degree in hand I headed to the great Pacific Northwest to find my fortune in the logging industry. I got a job involving helicopter logging, and lived in camps with ex-motorcycle gangs, murderers on the run, drug dealers, and country loggers. Drinking was possible only on the weekends. We worked hard and played hard. Marijuana always accompanied my drinking. I recall one weekend we went in to San Francisco, where I got extremely drunk and ran into some Moonies who were recruiting on the docks. They invited me to a meeting. I got into a massive fight in the hallway of a church and was bloodied up really bad. I ended up trying to get a prostitute and she also bloodied me up. I ended up passed out in shrubbery in front of a major hotel, with no clothes on, naked in a blackout. When I woke up in the morning there were 20,000 people on the sidewalk and a little boy said, "Mommy! Look at that bum.". I went back to the forest, and soon after that, headed back East—after ten years of logging.

I learned that my best friend, Pete, had died in a drowning accident—drunk—in New Jersey. This was one of the lowest points of my life. I headed to Northern Maine and started logging with the Canadian lumberjacks, but it just wasn't the same. I was trying to de-tox myself but found it impossible to go by a store that had beer in it without stopping to get drunk. I started having shakes and extreme headaches from alcohol.

I returned to RI, my home state, and at 29 years of age, called my parents from the side of the highway in East Greenwich to ask if I could live at their house while I got my act together. It didn't work. I went to the Narragansett Cafe in Jamestown every day and got extremely intoxicated. People in town avoided me. I had bad hygiene, a bad attitude and dreamed about killing people everyday. I was basically insane. One day, I jumped on a sailboat and berthed it off Nantucket, where I went ashore and got arrested three times in three days. The town judge told me to get off the island or he'd put me in jail for a year! I returned to Jamestown and stayed on another sailboat and drank from sun-up until sun-down. I ended up in Fall River, Massachusetts, somehow, and got into a fight with a biker, whom I threatened to kill. I also vowed loudly to cut the bar in half with my chainsaw. I was in big trouble with the law. I called my lawyer and he said it was either High Point Alcohol Rehab or the ACI.

I went to High Point, where I got so drunk I thought I was in college again studying alcoholism. My shaking was uncontrollable and I was starting to have liver problems. I got on the pink cloud real quick. I had not been sober since the age of 12 and I was 30. I was locked down for 30 days and started to learn about the program the day I got out. I went to the liquor store within ten minutes and started telling customers that alcohol would ruin their lives, and not to drink. I was kicked out of the store. I then decided to call a man I'd met in the program. He answered my call and told me to go to a meeting nearby and that he would meet me there. He is still my sponsor today.

I went by the Narragansett Cafe on my way to the meeting in Wickford, Rhode Island. I saw my friends drinking inside, and I learned later that while I was at that meeting one of my bar friends rolled over his pick-up truck on Beavertail Road and was thrown from the vehicle. The truck landed on his head. It was a turning point in my life. I went to a meeting every day for almost two years trying to learn how to live in sobriety.

My sobriety date is November 2, 1984. I have never had a relapse. I also have never smoked marijuana even though I had a good friend, Bill, who said 'with booze you loose but with dope there's hope'.

Other addictions have become prevalent in my life. I became a workaholic, starting a tree service and ending up becoming a nationally-known 'tree hugger', my smiling face splashed on the television screen and beaming from the pages of newspapers and magazine articles. It's hard to believe the turnaround. I have other addictions—food, Providence College basketball, laser sailboat racing, and, of course, the big one: sex!!! I could have sexual relations with my wife and ten minutes later want to have sex with the lady behind the counter at the coffee shop. This addiction has led to encounters with prostitutes, x-rated magazine shops and my newest addiction: computer sex. I have started attending meetings of Sexaholic Anonymous, because I believe it's my only way out.

One thing I have learned is that I don't like to hide my secrets any more. I remember how the fourth step used to intimidate me. But now I realize I'm as sick as my secrets. I just hit my 20th anniversary Nov. 2 2004 what a feeling!! Why Me?!! And what's in my future? I've always loved one day at a time and it is so easy to forget I'm one drink away from losing it all: the home on Jamestown, the lovely wife, my twin sons, my dog, my booming business, and my newfound self esteem. I have 20+ continuous years of sobriety, and have learned that only one out of 36 sober alcoholics have this achievement. I believe exercise has a lot to do with it. My job as an arborist keeps me outdoors every day of the year, so my other addiction is going in the forest after work and studying wildlife and ancient trees. I eat better than most and I sleep well when I have a normal week.

Five years ago I discovered and helped save an old-growth forest. It was a very spiritual experience. I have taken steps since then to save other old-growth forests and old-growth trees. I like to tell my mother, "Forest cathedrals are my church." I believe spirituality is a huge part of sobriety. I find complete peace working with trees and studying forests, including the creatures that live in the forest like black bears, fishers, bobcats, brook trout, ivory billed woodpeckers, moose, deer, coyotes and insects. There is a mountain in Maine, an old volcano called Mount Kineo that rises out of Moosehead Lake. I will leave Monday for another trip there to start the New Year on the right track.

Silence is golden.

The Twelve Steps of Alcoholics Anonymous

A.A. emphasizes in the chapter "How it Works" in the Big Book of Alcoholics Anonymous that the steps are "suggestions only" as a program for recovery, albeit life saving suggestions. [128]

Step One:

> *We admitted we were powerless over alcohol and that our lives had become unmanageable.*

Step one deals with the allergy to alcohol and addresses the physical aspect of the disease. Alcohol, once ingested, sets up a compulsive, insatiable craving for more. The vicious cycle of drinking, remorse and then more drinking has led many an alcoholic to his/her grave. Bill Wilson, the founder of A.A. writes in his own addiction story of the feelings associated with being beaten down by the obsession to drink: "No words can tell of the loneliness and despair I found in the bitter morass of self-pity. Quicksand stretched around me in all directions. I met my match. I had been overwhelmed. Alcohol was my master." (*The Big Book*, pg. 8) It is only through what the program calls the "gift of desperation" that the alcoholic is able to "hit bottom" and admit powerlessness over alcohol. Lack of power over alcohol ironically opens the way for the alcoholic to accept a power greater than himself for help with the obsession. The wreckage that active drinking causes in the life of the drinker and their loved ones is immense and devastating. Unmanageability asks the alcoholic to get out of the driver seat and be guided by the A.A. fellowship, one's sponsor and the principals of A.A. Powerlessness, when experienced rightly, is not hopelessness. On the contrary, it is the hope and grace that stem from surrendering one's willful, self-centered and self-destructive nature that gives the sufferer sustenance. We perceive that only through utter defeat are we able to take our first steps toward liberation and strength .[129]

Step Two:

We came to believe that a Power greater than ourselves could restore us to sanity.

Step two introduces the concept of a Higher Power and the spiritual nature of the recovery program. Being restored to sanity addresses the mental/emotional aspect of the disease. Coming to an understanding that excessive use and abuse of alcohol distorts our perception of reality is an important beginning to being restored to proper thinking. The A.A. program loosely defines insanity "as doing the same thing over and over again and expecting a different result." Surely the alcoholic operating under the illusion that he/she can control his/her drinking and that drinking can be "OK" is fitting that description. How Step Two works can be explained in the simple A.A. concept of—H.O.W.—Honesty, Open mindedness and Willingness:

> … honestly admitted that our defiance and self-will had almost destroyed everything in our lives, and that at running our own lives as active alcoholics, we were dismal failures. The open-mindedness to look at how a simple shift in perception away from ourselves and our wants and needs to a Higher Power, be it God or Group OF Drunks or Good Orderly Direction, had to produce better results. To have the willingness to follow the principals of the program, to abstain from drinking one day at a time, and to follow the guidance and suggestions of people in the program."[130]

The physical aspect of the disease is arrested by total abstinence, but the mental and emotional aspects of the disease are much more complex. Step Two begins the process of redirecting the alcoholic's distorted perception away from medicating reality to facing it squarely with the support of the fellowship.

Step Three:

We made a decision to turn our will and our lives over to the care of God as we understood him.

Lack of power over alcohol and the obsession to drink is turned towards a power greater than themselves. This is faith in action and is spelled out in the third step's prayer in the "Big Book" of Alcoholics Anonymous, "God, I offer myself to Thee- to build with me and to do with me as Thou wilt. Relieve me of the bondage of self, that I may better do Thy will. Take away my difficulties, that victory over them may bear witness to those I would help of Thy Power, Thy Love and Thy Way of Life. May I do Thy will always."[131] When Bill W. was asked if sobriety was all there was he replied, "No, sobriety is only the bare beginning; it is only the first gift of the first awakening. If more gifts are to be received, our awakening has to go on. As it does go on, we find that bit by bit we discard the old life—the one that didn't work—for a new life that can and does work under any condition whatever."[132]

Step Four:

We made a searching and fearless moral inventory of ourselves.

The writing of a personal inventory is taking stock of one's behavior and being accountable for the consequences. The philosopher Soren Kierkegaard once said, "We are condemned to live life forward, even though we can only view it backward." Taking a look at the "wreckage of our past" is an important step in freeing ourselves from its effects. Resentments towards people, places, and things are the focus of this step because it is believed that resentments are the number one killer of alcoholics. It is an emotion that no alcoholic wishing to stay sober can afford to foster.

Step Five:

We admitted to God, to ourselves and to another human being the exact nature of our wrongs.

Sharing our inventory with another person begins the process of being a part of the recovery program and the human race. The sense of isolation and self rationalization falls away and the opportunity to see the past as a tool to share with another suffering alcoholic takes its place. Shame and guilt in time are replaced by peace and acceptance. Self loathing can only heal when we bring it out into the light of forgiveness. Sharing the worst that is in us and the wrongs that we have done as active alcoholics, and realizing that we are not alone nor will we be rejected creates a release beyond description.

Step Six:

We were entirely ready to have God remove all these defeats of character.

While reading the inventory, a list of character defects and shortcomings emerges. This list is to be offered up to a Higher Power for healing and re-direction. Character defects are misdirected instincts that under the guidance of a Higher Power can be re-directed towards health and well being. Step Six speaks of becoming entirely willing, which in some cases, with certain defects, entails a process. Making a list and separating the characteristics that you are willing to give up from the ones that currently you are not willing to give up can be a good start.

Step Seven:

We humbly asked Him to remove our shortcomings.

This step deals with the concept of humility. Humility is being "right-sized" in the face of one's Maker and one's fellows. It is being grateful for the unmerited gifts given to each of us in life, and an appreciation for the Power behind them. Humility is knowing that God is the Creator, not you.

Step Eight:

We made a list of all persons we had harmed, and became willing to make amends to them all.

Step Nine:

We made direct amends whenever possible, except when to do so would injure them or others.

Steps eight and nine deal with the alcoholic's damaged relationships—personal, professional and spiritual. These steps are best approached with the guidance of a sponsor. Holding oneself accountable for past behavior without groveling, exaggerating, or self-condemning is no easy task, yet for the step to be healing and effective that challenge must be met. Compiling the personal inventory starts the process of paring away the emotional weights of guilt, shame, and self loathing. One of the promises in the Big Book of Alcoholics Anonymous is "We will not regret the past nor wish to shut the door on it."[133] Author Hugh Prather calls

Alcoholics Anonymous "the Berlitz course in spirituality". Anyone who has practiced these steps will surely agree.

Step Ten:

We continued to take personal inventory and when we were wrong, promptly admitted it.

The alcoholic is embarking on a lifetime of sober living and this on-going inventory helps the person in recovery to keep their "house clean and in order. Any build-up of resentments, illusions, or misdirected instincts can be dangerous for the person's sobriety. This inventory is a daily check in the present instead of the four step inventory which focuses on the past.

Step Eleven:

We sought through prayer and meditation to improve our conscious contact with God, as we understood Him, praying only for knowledge of His will for us and the power to carry it out.

The practice of prayer (talking with a Higher Power) and meditation (listening to a Higher Power) is a daily practice which allows the alcoholic to deepen his/her relationship with God. Author Scott Peck refers to the program of Alcoholics Anonymous as "The most powerful 'church' in this country ... Because it is the only program for conversion."[134]

Soon after Bill W read it for the first time at a General Service Organization meeting in 1940, the Serenity Prayer became the entreaty for recovering alcoholics nationwide. The author of the prayer was originally thought to be Dr. Reinhold Niebur of the Union Theological Seminary in New York City. Niebur wrote it down in its present form but admitted that it had most likely been around for perhaps centuries. In 1964 the office of A.A. was sent a clipping from the Paris Herald Tribune which credited the prayer to Friedrich Otenger an evangelical priest of the 18th century.[135] (AA, 2002) The debate may continue on who wrote this simple and yet profound prayer but the power of its words has no debate. It has helped millions of sober alcoholics in the rooms of A.A. all over the world for the last 65 years since the A.A. founder first read it. Many A.A. meetings open or close with these beautiful words,

God, grant me the serenity to accept the things
I cannot change,
The courage to change the things I can and,
The wisdom to know the difference.

Step Twelve:

Having had a spiritual awakening as a result of these steps, we continued to practice these principles in all our affairs.

In this step the program guarantees a spiritual awakening as a result of following the 12 steps. The founders of A.A. stated:

We have had a deep and effective spiritual experience which has revolutionized our whole attitude toward life, toward our fellows and toward God's universe. The central fact of our lives today is the absolute certainty that our Creator has entered into our hearts and lives in a way which is indeed miraculous.[136]

Dag Hammarsskjold wisely observed, "The longest journey is the journey inwards." After having traveled inward in steps 4 through 11 the 12th steps asks the alcoholic to then carry these principles out into everyday life. A life based on staying sober, one day at a time and in the practice of the steps of the A.A. program, coupled with assisting other alcoholics desiring to stop drinking and achieve sobriety are the basic tenets of A.A. It is said to be a program you give away to keep. Sharing the gift of sobriety by working with others and being of service to A.A. as a whole is reminiscent of the words of St. Ignatius of Loyola, "Let no one use anything as if it were his private possession." Staying sober is done in a community of support with the understanding that no one does it alone. The success or failure of any individual in the program affects everyone. Unity and service are the underpinnings upon which a lifetime of sobriety can be woven. Based on A.A.'s unprecedented success and longevity it is a concept that may be well worth adapting for all of us.

9

AN OUNCE OF PREVENTION

Relapse Prevention

It is said that progress is never in a straight line and sadly, for many recovering alcoholics, continuous sobriety can be elusive with periods of recovery followed by relapse into periods of drinking. It doesn't have to be that way, and if we can be keenly aware of the "warning signs" of relapse we can be well on our way to avoiding the pitfalls of active alcoholism. The "Big Book" of Alcoholics Anonymous refers to the disease as "cunning, baffling, and powerful". It is a disease that tells the sufferer that they do not have it. Denial, compulsivity and secrecy all conspire together to trick the alcoholic into thinking that maybe, just maybe, they can drink in safety. Anyone with experience in A.A. will tell you that no one comes back to A.A. happier and healthier after having drunk, on the contrary, they are often filled with shame and remorse and an overwhelming sense of dread about their future and their ability to once again achieve sobriety. Relapse does not have to be a part of a person's experience in sobriety. A.A. tells its members "just don't drink today—no matter what", and it is always *today*.

Here are some of the signs to look out for if you are in recovery.

Relapse Warning Signs

- Return to denial. This can come in the form of the nature of one's disease, behaviors that are self-destructive and not in keeping with a sober way of life, dishonesty, secrecy and addictive thinking patterns.

- Depressive mood, lack of self care and grooming, irregular sleeping habits, poor and/or irregular eating habits, apathy and loss of positive daily routine including not regularly attending A.A. meetings and sharing with A.A. sponsor and friends the truth about what is going on in one's life.

- Rejection of help, self pity, dissatisfaction with life, job and/or relationships, frustration with failures in one's life, lack of gratitude for sobriety and A.A.

- Anger, irritability, "leave me alone" and/or "I don't care" attitudes.

- Thinking about drinking, feeling jealous and/or angry of those who can drink, fanaticizing the glamour of drinking socially.

- Isolation in all areas of one's life. "Dry Drunk Syndrome" where all the internal and external feelings and behaviors mimic active alcoholism except for the ingesting of alcohol.[137] (Gorski, 1993)

Relapse Episode

The person resumes drinking and eventually the old drinking behaviors return. The feelings of self loathing and self pity overwhelm the addict often accompanied by feelings of loss of control of one's life which can lead in some cases to suicidal ideation. Once the disease is reactivated there is no guarantee that the person will be able to return to a sober way of living regardless of the length of time in sobriety prior to the "slip".

Relapse is a frightening fact for sober alcoholics, but it can be a healthy fear that keeps people vigilant in following their A.A. program and its guiding principles. Here are three case studies of women who each drank after periods of long-term sobriety (15 or more years) and were able to make it back to the rooms of A.A … In each case, warning signs of relapse manifested themselves, but the sufferers did not heed the signs. We human beings can learn from our own experience, or we can learn from the experience of others. The choice is ours:

Case Study:
Brenda's story

"I Was 15 Years Sober and a Certified Alcoholism Counselor When I Fell"

I grew up in a tight knit family of native Newporters who were in touch with numerous relatives on the island. Although we moved across the bay when I was five years old, we spent Sundays, holidays and summers back in Newport. We adhered to rules and traditions, such as arriving home from wherever we were by 5 in the afternoon to eat dinner together at 5:30, even though meal times with six children in the family were often tense situations. We took turns each week with chores like setting the table, clearing the table, washing dishes, and drying them (pre dishwasher). On Saturday mornings we could not go out until we each had dusted and vacuumed our bedrooms, changed the sheets on our bed, and cleaned one other room in the house.

We lived in a wonderful neighborhood with a pond to skate on in winter, and a huge swimming pool, tennis courts, and baseball fields for summer fun right at the bottom of our street. I can't recall ever hearing my parents' argue, which is not always a good thing because, as an adult, I had no experience with healthy conflict resolution. I also can't recall worrying about money, bills or other adult concerns when I was growing up, although my parents' consistently emphasized frugality.

I had a very low frustration level for delaying pleasure, so if my job was to dry the dishes, for example, and the other two siblings were taking their time clearing or washing, I would become angry. Saturday mornings were the pits because friends came ringing the doorbell and I couldn't go play, so I would apply half-measures and shove the clutter under the bed. I defied my parents in other ways as well, for example, by stealing money from them and shoplifting as a teenager because they would not buy me expensive things.

From the time I was six, until I was twelve, I was molested by an older cousin. His family had moved across the country and they came back to visit every other year. During those summer visits, we all stayed at my grandmother's house, so he had easy access to me. I felt 'bad" and blamed myself. My puberty was significantly impacted, since I was fearful of being "found out" and getting a negative reputation in high school. I vaguely remember abusing aspirin, especially during my periods, which were very painful. We had a male family doctor who told my mother I was being a "bit over the top" with my menstrual pain, but I remember it was as painful as childbirth.

At age 15 I began drinking with girlfriends, maybe once or twice a month on weekend nights. I LOVED that it turned my critical self-talk off, and allowed me to be at ease. I liked me! It was easier back then to get drugs rather than booze so I was introduced to pot, uppers, and downers, and diet pills became my first addiction. I loved the clarity and the focus that speed gave me. I did not know I could use other drugs to ease the crash of coming off the speed, and would often take uppers for 3 days straight before passing out. I spent the next nine years experimenting with drugs and alcohol, and became a daily user of drugs. I went from being an average B/C student to quitting high school my senior year because I had missed so many days of school. I returned to school during the last quarter and used speed to insure passable grades in order to graduate.

My disease brought me to new lows, which included new acquaintances, hard drugs, and frequent blackouts. I had arrests for shoplifting, drug possession, and was admitted to the hospital once for a suicide attempt (while using) and another time for de-tox/treatment. I was never arrested for DWI because I think it was not a known evil back then. The one time I could have shown probable cause for DWI, the local police officer was a kid I had gone to school with, and he brought me home. I knew I was out of control, but I thought I would grow out of this phase somehow—maybe if Mr. Right came along.

I'd lost jobs since my first one, due to my drug & alcohol use. I loved my first job in high school because the owner had bottles of speed & downers in his car and he would ask me to take his car for a fill-up at the gas station on Friday afternoons. After a while on this job, I began to steal from the register, and got fired after being employed two years there. I was unable to hold on to any job for more than six months during the next seven years because of my absenteeism. I was NOT a functioning alcoholic/addict.

In 1971, when I was 20, I sought help from my father. I told him I was using heroin, and he found a place that was newly-opened, called Caritas House. I had to go through detox at Chapin Hospital in Providence and then to the Institute of Mental Health, where Caritas House was originally housed. I was an emotional mess because I wanted to be accepted by others, but I associated with groups of people who were users and abusers. I was sincere in wanting to get straightened out emotionally, and so participated in group therapy and in one-on-one counseling to the best of my ability at that point in my life. I believed alcohol was still okay for me, though, and drank to get drunk regularly during my 2½ months in the program. My main drug was alcohol, with occasional tranquilizers

I did go to college that fall and knew to stay away from the "party people". I did very well during my first semester. During the second semester I started hanging out with people who liked to get high. By April I had quit school. The following January, I went to hairdressing school in hopes of getting my life together. I was doing well, and befriended a woman who lived in Newport with her husband. They found an apartment for me in their building, and I felt safe with them because they did not do drugs (he was a graduate of Marathon House). Once again, though, I was drinking.

After that great new start, I began hanging out with some of the gay guys at school and drinking martinis at their favorite hangout. Blackouts were frequent, and my survival tactic told me that a blackout while with these guys assured my safety from any sexual harassment. Once again I had quit school, had no job, and was on welfare. I was 23 years old and living in my little apartment with two cats. My friends on the second floor were no longer speaking to me because of my behavior while drunk, and my tolerance for alcohol was at an all time low. I would buy a six-pack of king-sized beer and maybe a pint of brandy if I had extra money. I could drink three beers and go into a blackout, or I would take Valium to help me become numb because the booze wasn't working. I felt suicidal, and after an overdose attempt, ended up in Newport Hospital. I was placed in their outpatient alcohol/Antabuse program, which operated very much like a methadone program, as I had to go there every day to get my Antabuse. AA meetings were a must in the treatment program, and I liked attending them. I was amazed at each day I went without drink or drugs. I did well for three months and then went out on a binge for nine days (four days were spent in a blackout), after which, I returned to meetings and outpatient treatment. I actively pursued AA meetings twice per day, and benefited from a sponsor, recovering friends, a home group, and the Twelve Steps.

I stayed sober from September 1975 through summer of 1990. I had been working as nationally-certified chemical dependency counselor in a 28-day rehab for almost ten years when I fell down a set of stairs and injured my back and neck (I never returned to work). It was weird timing because I was unhappy with the downward spiral the program seemed to be undergoing, yet I felt stuck about where to go next because I did not have my bachelor's degree. I was also at that point a single parent of two children, and was often tired, financially strapped, and lonely for a partner. My sponsor of 15 years had been having her own difficulties with physical ailments, and it did not occur to me to seek a new sponsor. With little guidance on my sobriety, serious pain and injuries from my fall, and prescriptions for pain pills, I was perfectly set up for a relapse.

I was diagnosed with cervical disease in May of 1990. I spent the next year attending meetings infrequently and going to different emergency rooms and doctors for pain medication. I kept all of this a secret except for telling one particular person. I picked up a drink in September of 1991, continued drinking, and for the next three years checked in to and out of rehab centers from New Hampshire to Florida. I would go back to meetings for a few weeks or for many months but I would not stay stopped. I would get sponsors, home groups, white chips, friends, and the return of my children to me and I was still not able to completely stop the relapse merry go round. I was arrested in 1993 for possession of cocaine and was held overnight in a Ft. Lauderdale lockup. I was in my early 40's and unique for finding myself in rehabs with younger people and/or people who had never experienced AA. I am an alcoholic who needs to feel a part of something and not alone.

The Grace of God re-entered my life in 1994 when I was once again placed in a long-term inpatient program in West Palm Beach. The difference this time is that I had a sponsor in this area with whom I had been working closely for eighteen months (twelve of those months I was sober). I was doing the steps, home group, friends and counselor. When I wanted to leave this program after a few weeks she would say things like "Your best thinking got you to where you are at now". I trusted her and I followed her suggestions. Three months later I left this program and moved into a Sober Apartment program owned by my counselor, and for the next year took direction from her and my sponsor. For the first time I did not have my children living with me upon leaving a treatment program. This was the most painful decision I've ever made. My family's suffering from my relapse is the most difficult thing for me to forgive myself for.

March 16, 1994 is my sobriety date. I have health issues today dealing with chronic pain due to initial cervical injury and fibromyalgia. I have one doctor who oversees my medical condition and my medications. I use acupuncture and neuromuscular therapy along with exercise, take vitamins and eat a wholesome diet to reduce the effects my health issues. I attend two or three meetings per week, and make a habit of going to at least the same two each week so I am familiar with and known by others. I speak at the meeting and/ or speak before or afterwards to others in the program. I have kept a dialogue about my thoughts with at least 1 or 2 other recovering women, including a former sponsor in Florida. I have just recently gotten a sponsor here in Rhode Island.

I pray each morning, asking to be kept away from drink and drugs and I thank God at night. I use my 40-minute ride to work to say the Third & Seventh Step prayers and to mentally list things for which I am grateful. I have used a therapist at various times and for short periods of time during the past eleven years. I have attended Ala-non throughout the past six years and read materials provided by these fellowships on a regular basis.

The three most important elements to my sobriety are friendships to whom I tell my Truth; meetings that teach me to laugh, cry, and be grateful; and contact each day with my Higher Power/God. I am truly grateful for each of my sobriety dates, for being attentive to my father while he was dying and being available to my sister, my brother and my son when they asked for help with their disease. I have been blessed many times in my life, and for the past four years, God has given me a chance at intimacy with a truly wonderful man. I was given another career and have been extremely successful at it, in spite of myself.

I am truly blessed with friendships I developed back in my early days of sobriety, and now have a history to look back on when I need it for my journey ahead.

Case Study:
Louise's Story:

"They Loved Me Back To Sobriety"

I grew up in a family whose main characteristic was a persistent sense of shame. I inherited it and developed shame of my own. My father was an alcoholic who had gotten sober when I was about three years old. My mother was long-suffering with him, as he was actually dry rather than sober. A successful restaurateur, he ruled over our family. I never felt that I could do enough to win his approval. Expectations for me were high but my performance invariably fell short of the mark, and there were reasons why this was so. One day, for example, my father asked me to carry a large watermelon to the house from the car. I was seven and I knew I couldn't do it, and I dropped it. The look on my father's face said what he was thinking. I simply could not measure up to his standards. When he passed away, everyone was relieved.

When I was thirteen I stole alcohol from my parent's liquor cabinet. It was Pinch scotch and the bottle was very attractive. I loved the feeling I got. I never drank socially. I believe my troubles with alcohol began when I drank that scotch, which was a troubled period for me. At that time, I was being molested by my older sister's boyfriend, who later became her husband. This was a terrifying burden and I told no one about it. I continued to steal alcohol and drink as often as I could.

I was very successful student and popular person in high school. When I began to drive, though, I drove drunk frequently. I hit parked cars and got away with that for awhile. I attended college and came home every weekend to drink. Alcohol was always on my mind.

I married my high-school sweetheart and moved to Boston, where he attended Harvard Medical School. I was teaching. I began to drink daily and soon became unable to function. I began to get Valium to help me over my hangovers. My main interest was to be able to drink, and I lived by the illusion that with enough effort I could control my drinking. My husband eventually divorced me because of my drinking. In the end, I lost that relationship, my job, and my self. I moved back home and continued to drink daily. I was unable to hold a job. I had hit bottom and I had nothing. It was this total deflation of ego and the pain it brought that broke the illusion that I could drink safely. My mother was very influential in my getting sober. I went through a detoxification program for 28 days and experienced a spiritual awakening. I stayed sober for 22 years.

During those years I attended AA regularly. After a year of sobriety I married a man who had thirteen years in AA, and we had been married for eight years when he suddenly died. I continued to stay sober with the help of AA and my relationship with God. I sponsored people and became a registered nurse. I married again. This relationship was difficult but passionate. One day, I inadvertently took some cough syrup for a legitimate cough. This triggered a love affair with the stuff. I secretly drank a whole bottle daily and thought I was getting away with it, even as my life began to erode. I withdrew from others, rationalizing that because there was no alcohol in the medicine, it was OK to continue taking it. This indulgence eventually cost me my sobriety. When my husband and I separated, I began a downward spiral that led me to the lowest point in my life. One day I bought alcohol and paid for it with a check, but have no recollection of this purchase at all. I was taken to Butler and diagnosed with bi-polar disease, and was prescribed Lithium. I had to tell the people that I sponsored that I had drunk. But this was not the end.

I could not stay sober. I was arrested several times for driving under the influence, and was on probation. I continued to drink, and although I sporadically went to meetings, I was lost. I drank again and was arrested for another DWI and was sent to the ACI for 10 days. Prior to this arrest I had secured a job in nursing and was stealing drugs occasionally. I came clean with that and received probation. After coming out of the ACI, I called my ex-husband to pick me up in Cranston. He and another friend took me to meetings for a year. They told me that they would love me back to sobriety until I was well enough to love myself. I stayed sober but I was miserable. It was almost a year before I began to warm up and clear up. Slowly, I began to be grateful and I made peace with my losses.

I still struggle with some aspects of myself and find that the phrase *Not my will but Thine be done* is very helpful. I pray each morning and evening. I am able to be a nurse again without impairment, and I do my best to be a good one. I am, however, struggling with food addiction which I believe stems from a deep-seated insecurity that I have never resolved. I deal with this insecurity and fear on a daily basis, but I apply the principles of AA to cope with it. I am also in therapy. I am still not happy with myself socially, and tend to withdraw from others and isolate myself, but I am holding on to the promises of AA and believe in the promise that fear of people will leave us. Despite all of the challenges, I now know a new happiness and a new freedom today.

I have been sober now for about four years. My sobriety date is December 8th. My attitude is one of gratitude and I believe that my sobriety is a gift. I do not want to loose it.

Case Study:
Ali's Story

"I Put My Daughters in Foster Homes so that I Could Drink"

I was adopted as an infant, and always felt I was chosen by my parents, and so had no special interest in my birth parents. I grew up a happy kid who loved to play, draw, and read. My dad was from a line of naval officers, and his career was with the Navy as well. As a child, I did well in school until we moved to France when I was 10. My mother put us in a French Catholic school so that we could learn the language. This was demoralizing and humiliating as I was placed in 4th grade instead of 6th, and I was considered a total oddball—and a protestant! My only sibling, a sister two years younger than I, attended the school, too, but we didn't see each other. We really hated going to that school.

The first time I drank was at a christening for a French family. My parents were asked to be godparents and wine was served. The waiters kept filling the glasses, and I kept drinking. I loved it. I spoke French, danced, and felt fabulous. After that, whenever my parents had cocktail parties, I would help clear up and sip the dregs of their friends' unfinished drinks. When my mom got hepatitis (from eating tainted seafood) we started going to the American school in Paris which was another shock because I had grown accustomed to a small independent, private school through Grade 5. The new school was confusing, and I felt a lot of social pressure fit in, and an inability to do so—or to be liked. I stopped being really interested in school and became totally boy crazy, as well as obsessed with movie stars and American music. We left Paris for the south of France when I was in 7th grade.

I excelled in the new school, but that summer I was 13 and took up drinking with a vengeance. I had a lot of strange physical encounters with older teenage boys and many blackouts. I drank whatever was being passed around. I thought I was living an exciting life—sneaking out and staying out. My parents were out or away a lot and left us with a French housekeeper who I know today to be an alcoholic. I never saw any drunkenness or inappropriate behavior from anyone in my family—other than me! When we came back to the States, my parents were beginning to worry about me and so sent me to a college prep boarding school. I got kicked out for smoking cigarettes. After two years, I was asked back. They said I was not taking advantage of the opportunities I was being offered, and told me about my IQ and my potential. But by then I just wanted to get some beer and go to the graveyard and drink. I had boyfriends from town and lost my virginity when I was 15. I had no boundaries about my body, no self-respect for it, and detached myself mentally from it. I drank whenever it was available or whenever I could get someone to buy alcohol for me. The summer my mom took me to see the public high school I would be attending for 11th grade in Washington, DC, something in me snapped and I knew I couldn't go to that school. I was pregnant, and got married within 6 months. I was drunk when I got pregnant and continued to drink throughout my pregnancy. My daughter was born when I was 17. I became pregnant again within 2 months after the baby's birth. My doctor told me that breastfeeding was natural birth control. I told her I couldn't have another baby but she said, "Nonsense you're married now." I fell into a depression but didn't know it at the time. Within the next year and a half, I had given birth to my second daughter, gotten arrested for pot possession, taken up with my husband's best friend, and put my daughters in foster homes. I then signed papers to give them up for adoption. I made this decision during a time I was drinking, smoking pot, taking LSD or doing whatever I wanted. So the next 7 years were a downhill spiral.

I lived in a lot of interesting places—the West Indies, for example—and had fun jobs—working on charter sailing boats and such, but I was a wreck inside. I kept going from one relationship to the next, but nothing or no one ever fixed me or made me feel better. Whenever I thought about my past, I hated myself. I could not accept myself, let alone forgive myself. I got into more drugs, heroin, and cocaine. I would really try anything, but I never shot dope because I felt I had to have some standards for myself. I was in love with a junkie at one time, and sat by him as he shot up many times. Maybe it helped me feel better about myself that I never shot up.

A few boyfriends later, I hit bottom. I had a bad car accident and totaled my car and ended up in the hospital. When I got out and had the ability to move, I moved to Rhode Island. Within 6 weeks, my new life was like the disastrous one I had left in Annapolis, Maryland. I had truly hit bottom. I called AA. I went to my 1st meeting—identified—and felt hope for the 1st time that maybe I could find a new life. I got a sponsor and became very involved in the program. It took me the first year to stop doing drugs, though I couldn't get the connection between the obsession and the compulsion.

When I was addicted, it was as though someone else was living my life. I did not do what I intended to, and all my good intentions, hopes, and dreams were forgotten for the "high" I would do anything to experience. I would spend all my time and energy getting high, and never finished high school or held a real job. I was undependable, unpredictable and disappointing, mainly to myself, as well as untrustworthy and paranoid and moody to others. I thought about suicide a lot and was cynical of life and filled with contempt for happiness of others. I was truly dead inside, a consequence of drinking from the ages of 13 to 26—before I found AA.

AA brought me back to life. In its hands I cried and laughed and started to feel again. I got sober by being in close contact with a sponsor and by going to two meetings a day for the first year. I had to join a group and become active with that group. I had to give out my phone number and give rides to girls who didn't have cars. I had a sponsor who had been through a 12-step halfway house and she was very strict. She was also incredibly generous in giving me a lot of time. As I began to feel better, I started to do things my way. I didn't get the connection between my personal life and AA. So I went out with someone who drank and used drugs. I smoked hash, ate mushrooms, and finally did coke with him—the only drug I swore I couldn't do safely, and I got pregnant again, by a man who had gotten sober briefly, but who didn't want to get married or be a father. I was all set with an appointment for an abortion when an AA friend asked me to try to do some writing about this pregnancy. The writing made it clear that I wanted and loved that baby and believed I could be a good mother. Now I had a program and was clean and sober. I stayed pregnant, and soon began a new relationship with a man 8 years younger than I, who was also in AA. He wanted to get married, adopt my baby and build a life together. I wasn't sure I was ready for all that, but he gave me an ultimatum and as I was afraid to lose him and become a single parent, so I agreed to marry him. I loved many things about him but also knew it was a mistake to marry him. He adopted my daughter, and two years later, we had twins. We were married for 12 years. I had stopped going to meetings when we moved, because it was easier to be home with my family than to go out and have to make new friends. We became isolated and only had a few couples as friends. We didn't mean to put AA out, but it just happened. I didn't think of drinking, but I let the steps slip out of my life in reverse. I didn't carry the AA message, and had no spiritual practice or reliance on God. I blamed my husband for my problems, as I thought him a perfectionist and very controlling. I never learned to stand up for myself. Early in our marriage when I had tried to make a decision for myself, he became physically angry and frightened me. I backed down and became a perfect, submissive wife, but an obsessive one.

I continued smoking off and on, and developed an eating disorder. I was a compulsive overeater and exerciser and obsessed about how I looked, how the house looked, and how the garden looked. I did not look within. I just hoped everything would be OK. My husband left us after twelve years, over a money issue. During our marriage, we would pay off our credit card debt annually through monetary gifts from my father. At one point, my husband wanted to take out a second mortgage, but I refused to sign the papers. I knew that any big chunk of cash would not solve our financial problems because we had been continually living beyond our means. I had all the material advantages growing up, and he had none, so the mortgage loan meant he could finally get some of the things he wanted, but this was the first and only time I said no to him. Within a couple of months he asked for a divorce. Those proceedings took two years and were horrible in terms of his behavior to the children (totally abandoning them without giving us even a phone number to reach him) financial costs, and fear. My father rescued me financially so I could keep the house. I returned to a few AA meetings.

The meetings gave me a sense of relief, but I didn't really share honestly my extreme pain and feelings of abandonment. Instead, I got into a string of inappropriate short term sexual relationships with men in AA. I felt taken advantage of by one of them, and in turn I took advantage of someone else. All of this behavior made me feel shameful, but I also enjoyed the attention and the attraction these men showed me. I was craving love and attention. At this time, though, I neglected my children's needs for attention. Keeping the house, having clean clothes and providing food seemed to me to be enough. I got involved with one man who was very active in AA and my meeting attendance increased, but I never really self-examined. I was preoccupied with trying to figure out what to do with my life after the divorce.

As far as career changes during this time, I had sold my business and exercise studio, and couldn't handle the pressure of real estate sales any longer. I had returned to waitressing and wanted to start attending college again. I had to get my GED even though over the years I had accumulated over 60 college credits. I did get accepted into a two-year program for Physical Therapy Assistant. At that time, too, I broke up with the nice AA guy and started up with another man who was sober but who didn't go to meetings. That lasted a year, during which I further neglected my children. They, in turn, began to have difficulties of their own, but my self-centeredness and lack of any grounded program of recovery kept me from helping them. At that time, life threw me a curve.

My dad got killed crossing a street in Florida. I couldn't stand the painful feelings that resulted. I immediately went back to smoking cigarettes and after being the strong one for the rest of the family, I started smoking pot within two months after the death of my father. I went to a few meetings but I never told the truth. I justified and rationalized and the progression downhill was steady. I increased my smoking from one night a week to every day. I avoided contact with my mother in order to get home to relax and smoke. I became very secretive and continually lied to myself. I planned and took a ten-day trip to France. Prior to setting off, I went to several meetings because I was afraid I would be tempted to drink in France. At the meetings, I "told on myself" but did not admit that I got high.

After my father's death, I had become involved with a man 20 years younger than I who was a chronic pot smoker. Part of my relapse involved being in a very slippery place when I was most vulnerable, i.e., grieving for my father. This continued for 3 ½ years.

I had enjoyed enough accomplishments to convince myself I was doing fine, including earning a Bachelor's degree in physical therapy. That seems to me now only an outward achievement. Inside, I was blocked with self-centered justifications and lies. I had not had a drink or substitute for 17 years when I picked up the pot. One night a girlfriend asked what I was waiting for after I had talked about the changes I needed to make to get my life together again. When she left, I smoked a joint, but strangely I didn't get high. I felt a sense of impending doom as I've never felt before. I feared I might get arrested, lose my license to practice physical therapy, lose my job, or end up reported in the newspaper. Thinking about all I had to lose filled me with fear and humiliation. The next day I broke up with that man, got rid of the dope, and went back to meetings.

I have been clean and sober for 8 ½ years now, July 19, 1996 is my new date. Changing the date was big but I had to be totally honest. I quit smoking about 18 months into my recovery because I finally got sick and tired of being owned by nicotine, whether cigarettes, gum or the patch. I feel well, although I can still get in trouble with food, though I understand when I'm trying to use a substance to make me feel better.

I now attend 3–5 AA meetings a week, sponsor 5 women, and have a sponsor myself. I don't minimize anything any more. I journal every day, pray and meditate, and have joined a church during the last year. I exercise daily through walking, yoga, golf, or swimming. I limit coffee to two cups a day. I have sleeping problems, so I take hot baths. I limit TV to maybe 5 hours a week. I thrive on routine. I limit sugar and white carbohydrates for mental balance. My ex-husband died of alcoholism in a drunk driving motorcycle accident and I was able to be there for my children. I was able to go to counseling to deal and work through the grief I felt for his loss as well as the loss of my father. I go to step meetings and have taken a thorough 4th step. I met and married a fellow AA after a lengthy courtship. I am learning to think things through, ask for help, and not react on impulse. I am filled with gratitude for the many blessings in my life, for each experience, whether of joy or pain, to learn a lesson from. I am being drawn closer to my higher power and to other people. I have returned to school to study painting, resurrecting a teenage dream. I am close to my children and have shared my story, all of it, with them. It's all I have, but it's everything.

These stories hold powerful lessons, but many relapses do not have happy endings. As the Big Book of Alcoholics Anonymous reminds us, "Once an alcoholic, always an alcoholic. Those commencing to drink after a period of sobriety are, in a short time, as bad as ever. If the alcoholic is to cease drinking, there can be no reservation to quit entirely, no lurking notion that someday he/she will be immune to alcohol."[138]

10

A SPIRITUAL AWAKENING

Alcoholism is not overcome by extraordinary will power; it is overcome by a complete surrender to a Higher Power through an admission of powerlessness.

This spiritual relationship with a power acknowledged as greater than the individual, and moreover, the quality of that relationship, is ultimately the only defense against the first drink. This is clearly spelled out in A.A.'s Big Book when it says, "The alcoholic at certain times has no effective mental defense against the first drink. Except in a few rare cases, neither he nor any other human being can provide such a defense. His defense must come from a Higher Power."[139]

The Spiritual Awakening

The spiritual awakening is promised in the twelfth step of the program, but what really is it? Do you wait to see a burning bush or flashing lights or Heavenly beings? This might be the experience of some and surely the founder of A.A., Bill Wilson's experience was miraculous by anyone's account, but most experience a gradual change. "Most of our experiences are what the psychologist William James calls the "educational variety" because they develop slowly over time."[140] In a letter to Carl Jung, a longtime supporter of Alcoholics Anonymous Bill Wilson writes, "My release from the alcohol obsession was immediate. I knew I was a free man…. In the wake of my spiritual experience, there came a vision of a society of alcoholics, each identifying with and transmitting his experience to the next-chain style…. This concept proved to be the foundation of such success as Alcoholics Anonymous has since achieved."[141] Wilson always said it was a God-given program; therefore a God of your understanding can lead you to sobriety, safety and a new purpose for your life—if you will only let it.

Spiritual Surrender

Sober alcoholics often recall a moment of complete demoralization, what AA calls "hitting bottom". The moment is filled with despair and hopelessness because the alcoholic sees for the first time without any denial the truth about his/her drinking. The lies fall away, the fantasies, the glamour and the bright lights and all that is left is a feeling of impending doom and powerlessness. In that moment each person said a prayer—not a religious prayer filled with faith, but a desperate prayer filled with fear. The total surrender that brought about a willingness to do anything to escape the horror of an alcoholic death strangely and miraculously led to a solution. Such a prayer was uttered when Ray realized that he had spent the evening nurturing his drink instead of caring for his very ill son—forgetting to give him the much needed medicine he promised his wife he would not forget when she left the house for a few hours.

Case Study:
Ray's Story

"The Easier, Softer Way"

I was born in Providence, RI in 1925 during my father's final year at Harvard Law School. In 1928, we moved to a suburb of Chicago where my paternal grandfather was rector of a large Episcopal church and my maternal grandparents lived as well. My two sisters were born there. We were brought up in a very loving home; however, disaster was on the horizon. In November of 1938, my mother died very suddenly and the family was shattered. My father started drinking quite heavily in his grief. I was in my teens at the time and I was very concerned about him and the possibility that he might lose his job at the University where he was teaching law. Somehow, he managed to hang on and when the U.S. got actively into World War II, he got a commission in the Army and went to Washington D.C. In the meantime, during my Junior/Senior years in High School, I occasionally had a beer or two, but not enough to get drunk. I used to think that it enhanced my piano playing when some of my friends and I had jam sessions.

It wasn't until I got out of Marine Corps boot camp that I first got drunk. I got very sick and I blacked out. I needed to be able to handle my duties, so the drunks were rather few and far between.

My father remarried while I was overseas and his drinking became more normal again. He, fortunately, was not an alcoholic. It was a different story for me, however.

After the War II, I went to college on the GI Bill. My drinking and general hell-raising made a mess of things. I left after three semesters before I got tossed out. This, of course, went over big with my family. I knew that my drinking was a problem. I hated blacking out and the hangovers, but I wasn't about to accept being an alcoholic.

After leaving school I managed to get a job in the corporate purchasing department of a large multinational corporation in New Jersey. I wanted to hang on to the job so I didn't drink while I was working. I confined my drinking to the evenings. I didn't drink on Sundays, as I usually used that day to recover and get ready for work on Monday.

I started to hate the way I was living and I suffered periods of severe depression. I tried all the tricks in attempting to control my drinking. I would stop for short periods, but couldn't stay stopped. I didn't know it at the time, but the progression of the disease had set in years earlier. I was hooked. I hated banging around from pillar to post and staring at a gloomy future.

In 1950, I met a wonderful young lady. We fell in love and were married in 1951. Little did she know what she was getting herself into. She didn't know how much I drank. I, however, thought this was precisely what I needed to get out of the awful rut I was in and was determined to be a good and responsible husband. Things went along pretty well for a while. I was progressing on the job, and was by this time a buyer. The "business lunch" had become an almost daily affair with two or three drinks beforehand. I was what is called a functioning alcoholic and full of denial. I hadn't gotten into any serious public difficulty, although I was pretty good at making an ass out of myself at social affairs.

During the sixties, we had five children. The first two, a girl and a boy, were adopted, and then we had our first biological baby who was to be with us only three months when he died of SIDS. Needless to say, this was a heart-wrenching event. Two more children were born, another girl and boy. I loved my family dearly and strove to be a good husband and father, but the disease was progressing. We were very active in our church, yet this didn't seem to have much of an impact on my problem. I was becoming paranoid and was having horrendous anxiety attacks. I thought that I was losing my mind at times. I had become very erratic in my behavior, lovingly collected and engaged one minute and breathing fire in the next. It's a wonder that I still had a family and my job. To feed my denial, I never had a DWI, I was never hospitalized for alcoholism, never lost a job, and have never been a patient in a rehab.

During the summer of 1975, I was in terrible shape emotionally. My house of cards was starting to collapse and the possibility of losing everything was becoming very real. Our youngest son had serious health problems and was being given medicine at regular times. On the evening of August 4th, my wife had to go to a meeting and left me in charge with specific instructions concerning his medication which was of life-saving importance. After the children were in bed, I settled down in the den to watch TV and, of course, I had poured myself a drink. When my wife came home, I was still in my chair with a drink in my hand. She asked me if I had given our son his medicine. Fortunately, I was not plastered and I realized—to my horror—that I had not given my son his medication, and that it was way past time. My wife looked at me with complete disgust and said that she could never again leave me with the children and stormed upstairs. I sat there with the guilt welling up within me and was completely disgusted with myself. That was the last straw. The house of cards had crashed. I went into the kitchen and threw the rest of my drink into the sink and went up to bed. I lay in bed totally distraught and knowing that I was at the point of no return. I uttered the most honest prayer I have ever uttered: "God help me!!!" It was then that the miracle started to happen. An amazing sensation started to come over me. It started at my feet and worked its way up completely enfolding me. I felt a presence. The feeling was overwhelming, and I broke down. Tears of awe and wonder filled my being, and I felt totally calm and serene. I woke my wife and told her that I was going to go to AA the next day. I had very little knowledge of AA, and, like most of us who enter the fellowship, had erroneous, preconceived ideas. I did find a meeting in the next town on August 5th and have been going ever since. I believe that on that fateful night in 1975 the obsession was lifted from me by the grace of God.

I have never had a desire to drink since, and it has been twenty nine years, one day at a time. I was never involved with drugs other than alcohol.

I was able to give my employer twelve years of sober employment before I retired after forty years in 1987. I have had no need for anything other than AA to keep me grounded in sobriety and I am totally grateful to God and the Fellowship, and to my dear wife of 53 years for being able to stick it out during those unhappy years.

Life has been good in sobriety. It is wonderful to have a loving family, all of whom are sober. The only other alcoholic in our family is our oldest daughter and she has been sober for twenty five years. I have remained very active in the Fellowship and usually attend five meetings a week, and I have found the twelve steps to be indispensable for growth in sobriety. Surely, it is the easier, softer way.

Marilyn's story has a similar theme. She was busy living the good life and alcohol and alcoholic relationships played important roles in such a life. It was not until she had finally found her "soul mate' that the threat of her drinking and her out-of-control behavior was seen in its true light. The fear of losing his precious love led to an epiphany. She has been sober ever since that moment—some 271/2 years now. Here is how her story unfolds.

Case Study:
Marilyn's Story

"Gracious Living"

I began drinking in high school with my first boyfriend and with friends of his who were a bit older than he was. They drank, so I thought that was the thing to do. My earliest drinking experiences involved getting drunk and throwing up, but I persisted and learned the knack of it. From the beginning I had hangovers, but it never occurred to me to stop drinking. In my attempts to control, I made it a point to drink only on Friday and Saturday nights (in the early years) because the mornings-after were so awful.

I was angry much of the time after I married that high school sweetheart. He stayed out late drinking and didn't take me along, and then wouldn't call me while he was out. Years later I realized that this feeling of being neglected was part of my fury. He didn't want alcohol in the house, so on top of feeling ignored, I thought I was missing out on a lot of fun as well.

My second husband was a different type of drinker. "This is more like it," I said to myself. He was elegant and had a complete bar in his bachelor pad overlooking the San Fernando Valley. He and his friends entertained at home with dinner parties, bracketed with a stream of before-and-after-dinner drinks—the appropriate wines flowing freely in between. I thought it quite the "gracious living" life style, with daily cocktails part of the routine. It took me a while to realize my handsome husband was passing out, not merely falling asleep, each night after our late dinner.

The second divorce I blamed on his infidelity.

When I met my third husband, I thought, "This is it—My problems are over." I assured myself, "We are soul mates—no doubt about it." We drank together and thought the good times would never end. But a funny thing happened: whereas in my previous marriages, it always seemed I was in control and they (the husbands) drank too much, this time it was different. To my dismay, I found that my drinking was out of control. I behaved badly and found my "perfect' relationship beginning to unravel. I arrived at the demoralizing knowledge that I was alcoholic and that I was powerless. That summer of 1977 was pure hell. I couldn't stop drinking and knew that I was destroying myself and any hope of a happy life.

The fall came during the night when I was, to put it honestly, shit-faced drunk, yet feeling stone-cold sober at the same time. I knew I was doomed. It was the dark night of the soul. I heard myself cry out 'God help me." A peace came over me that I've heard sometimes described as an "epiphany" and I was able to fall asleep. When I awakened the next morning I knew I would never have to drink again.

Having said that, I also must tell you I had a horrible fear that the obsession could come back, for I knew without a doubt I was, am, and always will be … powerless over alcohol.

I called a woman I knew who had stopped drinking and she told me that although she hadn't needed it, she knew where there was a noon meeting of Alcoholics Anonymous. I went to that meeting. I bought the big book and picked up pamphlets. I have never had a drink since that day, September 21, 1977. I have taken the steps, and do a quick 'tenth' by way of reviewing my day when I settle down for a night's sleep, and I still aim for seven to ten meetings a week.

Happy note: that dear husband number three came to the program, also, and we enjoyed a remarkably happy marriage until he died, sober, in 1986.

Alcoholics Anonymous is the best thing that ever happened to me. Today I enjoy harmonious relationships with family members by practicing these principles in all my affairs to the best of my ability.

Sept 21, 1977 is my sobriety date. I have not relapsed. I have experienced periods of depression, but they were times when depressing things were going on. I have come to accept the full spectrum of emotions and am willing to go through them.

It is my belief that it is mentally healthy to feel depressed in the face of depressing events. I no longer think that I should somehow be entitled to go through life without experiencing sadness, grief, or depression. I do NOT think that peace of mind comes in a pill or capsule. I do not think that peace of mind, or serenity, is synonymous with "happiness." It is paradoxical, but I have experienced, in sobriety, the possibility of feeling serene and sad at the same time.

I calculate that I have been sober now for as long a period as I drank—27 years drinking—starting at age sixteen—and 27 years of continuous sobriety, from age forty-three to seventy.

Holy smokes! Time flies when one is having fun (and when one *isn't*.)

11

A FAMILY DISEASE

Stories of Family Alcoholism and Abuse

Both of the following stories illustrate the role that alcoholism can play in a family, and ways active alcoholism often leads to other forms of abuse. Alcoholic homes are filled with family secrets. Children in these families are told, "Don't talk, don't trust, don't feel". (Reddy, p.7). The child has to carry the burden of these conditions often while being physically, emotionally, and, in some cases, sexually abused. It is no wonder that many of these children turn to alcohol themselves for comfort and coping. In the following two stories these two women were raised in such homes.

Case Study:
Lee's Story

"Just in the Nick of Time"

My childhood was pretty scary. My earliest memory was being in a bathtub with my stepfather, and my mother was very angry because he had braided my hair into many pigtails making me look like "pick-a-ninny". I was not feeling safe because he was drunk. They both drank. Mom was left home to care for us kids and Dad was out drinking in bars. Left all alone my mother became very aloof, sickly, and very, very unhappy. This was made worse when she had to have a complete hysterectomy at age 27.

My home life was a nightmare. My stepfather, Herbie, had a drinking problem as well, and Mom's angry responses to his not coming home on time, resulted in violent fights. The police would show up and we would flee in middle of the night to a motel. Most weekend nights found me going to bed, the family's sharpest butcher knife under my pillow, and me lying awake for hours in terror that I would have to kill Herbie. As a result of all the stress, I was a terrible student, unable to concentrate, and apt to dissolve into tears in the middle of class, thereby mortifying myself and getting labeled as a "discipline problem". I was eight and a half years old and would be shaken from sleep routinely for the 2 am feeding of a new baby brother. The nights Dad stayed home, I would sit in the dark on the outside stoop while he drank his hidden beer and whistled "Don't Fence Me In". Then I would listen to his babbled nonsense.

We lived near an airport, and I remember sitting for hours praying that my "real" Dad would somehow be miraculously "found"—despite his MIA status—come home, and rescue me from this never-ending nightmare. He had been killed three months before I was born.

Lucky for me, we moved to beautiful Wickford, Rhode Island, and by this time I was new in town, blonde, and pretty. I was moving out from under the violence at home by being mobile with lots of friends. A new nightmare was now unfolding, however: I was playing "dodge 'em' with my stepfather. At night I would come home to a darkened house where the only visible thing was the glow of Herbie's cigarette. Scurrying to my room, I was forced to listen to his tirade of filthy accusations about things he imagined I was doing with boys—all of it untrue, as I was a good kid.

Those were frightening nights, and I never felt safe until the daylight. At 16, I started to experiment with alcohol—just to fit in. My reaction was always the same: tears, or a maudlin disposition. Nevertheless, those years in Wickford were a dream. It was a small town and we had the sophistication of the Navy kids and a nearby university—so we drank beer on weekends. One night, I was riding with a car full of kids and the driver veered off the road and smashed into a tree. I suffered a broken back. This happened practically in front of my home, but it wasn't my parents that rode in the ambulance to the hospital with me, it was my friend Susan. My parents were just a mess and too drunk to care. I could not wait to get away from them and get control of my life. I swore I would never, ever, be like them.

Within a month of graduating from high school, my stepfather dropped dead from a major coronary. He was only 42. My family was plunged into enormous despair. My mother was inconsolable. I had qualified for a college scholarship as a result of my real dad's death and my high IQ, but I was unable to pull it off in the end. As much as I wanted to get away from home, I was too frightened to follow my friends off to college. I wanted security more than anything, so I married the boy who took me to my high school proms. Both of us merely took each other hostage so we could get out from under the suffocating control of my alcoholic family and his overly religious household. We had children right away and the stresses were enormous. We were children having children. Weekend drinking helped me to relax, or so I thought. I always got as drunk as I could. I was desperately seeking oblivion from all my new found constrictions. I had a nervous breakdown and went on medication that I didn't think helped at all. Shortly after that, my Mom died at 44, and I suffered another total breakdown. Now I was on big-time meds that rendered me a zombie similar to Jack Nicholson's portrayal of the post-lobotomy patient in "One Flew Over the Cuckoo's Nest". I started the daily drinking of wine and beer, as this was the only thing that gave me hope. I drank in the mornings and throughout the day until I was able to sleep at night, but always woke up around 2AM, loaded with paralyzing fear. It was a living nightmare, with the only hope found in the momentary relief that alcohol delivered. Anxiety attacks and agoraphobia followed me everywhere, but mostly to the boundaries of my yard for I could not go anywhere else. I felt certain I would embarrass myself with my anxieties playing out publicly if I left home. I simply could not function. I also felt horror and disappointment in knowing I could not be the energetic and focused mother and member of the community I had dreamed I would be someday. I was desperately afraid I might be one of those mothers who would harm her children (like Andrea Yates, the Texas mother who, in 2001, drowned her children.) I, however, lived only for my children at this time, and would not force them to live with the legacy of pain that my suicide would bring them, thank God.

The horror of my ways went on for seven years before things got slightly better, but I was to drink alcoholically for ten years altogether. I could never be comfortable in public with my drinking, as I was still emoting, and I feared I would be a "blurter" with terrible emotional repercussions in the form of just being so ashamed of who I was at my deepest level. The fear of going "public" with my thought that I might be really crazy—coupled with my agoraphobia—kept me primarily in the home. I had married a man totally incapable of helping me on any level. He was doing his best to survive in the quagmire of our life together. Despite having been voted most popular, best personality, and friendliest in my high school class, I had alienated everyone as a result of my mental illness and my drunken outbursts. I was totally alone. Thank God for booze, it really did keep me alive till the day it no longer worked and I was plopped into the halls of Alcoholics Anonymous.

AA was the greatest thing that ever happened to me. I loved it right from the beginning. I had never identified with anyone in any of the group therapy situations in which I had found myself, but those sessions had set the stage for understanding the steps of AA. It all made sense to me staring at the steps during my second or third meeting. I felt so connected! What a relief at finally finding out what was "wrong" with me and my family. I believed right from the beginning that I had been hardwired with the disease. Now I felt such real hope, and not the kind that was manufactured in my brain from the bottle. Now I would be "OK". I was safe at last, just in the knick of time, as they used to say. I got a very strict sponsor who also had a lawyer for a husband. He helped us with business problems, which were truly terrible. She was a godsend for me, as I was awfully self-willed. My fear of her, though, motivated me to do things that kept me from going out and getting drunk. I joined a stand-up group and we traveled around the three states speaking and carrying the message of AA. This was great, and had contributed to a change my husband made from being a passive husband to an active parent. I was now out every night at a meeting in a car loaded with recovering people who would tell me my agoraphobia and anxiety would go away if I didn't drink, if I prayed, and if I went to AA meetings. I believed everything anyone told me and I truly began to bloom with the fervor seen in charismatic congregations or Evangelical missions. Finally, I felt special—anointed even, and hopeful for the "perfect" life I had desired.

August 20, 1979 is my anniversary date. I am now 60 years old. I have never relapsed, due, I believe, to the actions I take on a daily basis to treat my three-fold disease: I start my days on my knees telling God I am powerless over booze, asking to be restored to saner thinking, and establishing a willingness to turn my life over to His direction for one day. I ask God to not let me drink (or overeat compulsively) for this one day. I also ask for a grateful heart and to cause no harm for that day. I go to five or six AA meetings a week, one Al-Anon meeting a week, and one FA (food addicts) meeting a week. I talk weekly to my sponsor, a Harvard-trained behavioralist, who like me, craves honest conversation about what events occur in our lives and our reactions to those situations. We cry or roar with laughter over our antics. Those conversations free me from the self-doubts that creep in during the week. We are in the middle of yet-another fifth step and it is a painful/illuminating experience. This is the action I take for the emotional aspects of my disease. I have had a lot of therapy, but I find my relationship with my sponsor to be the most satisfying element with respect to maintaining awareness, sustaining growth, and accepting my own humanity and that of those I love and encounter.

I've tried using meditation techniques, but it seems my type-A personality just doesn't slip into that the level of relaxation and sense of well-being anymore. In addition, I've given up my weekly church-going as part of the process of treating my spiritual needs. I used to claim I was going to church to thank God for my blessings. Really, though, I was going to cover my bases, as I was afraid that I was not doing "enough" for God to keep me sober and he would strike me "drunk" if I didn't go. Also, I wanted to show members of my community what an upstanding member I was, just in case they had heard I was an alcoholic. That is me, always trying to redeem myself from the shame of being me or "earning my keep" (with God) because as a child I felt like such a burden to my parents. As a sales rep who travels long distances, I must say that I feel closest to God when I'm traveling. During these times, I am hyper-aware of nature as He created it and I experience a lot of awareness about my life while on the road. Perhaps I've had to let the pendulum swing a bit and discover that God loves me, and not because I'm "good".

So now I'm 25+ years sober and while I maintain a heavy meeting schedule, the number is partly due to the loneliness I feel inside. My life has a melancholy cast that perhaps is due to the remains of childhood, losses of loved ones, menopause, and also to the new set of expectations that were created when I joined AA. Having been a person who always wanted to be "saved" by people, places, or things, AA was the answer to my lifelong yearning. I listened carefully at those early speaker meetings, especially to the part about "life getting so good that just when you think it can't get any better, it does". I bought into that and subconsciously my belief system tells me that since I'd been "rescued". I'd draw a pass on the other problems ordinary folks had because after all, I'd lost three parents, an infant, had two nervous breakdowns and was now an alcoholic! I thought that because now I'm on a mission for God, I would coast through life with my "shit happens" credit card prepaid! So when I feel lonely or blue, I think I'm doing something wrong (or not doing enough), rather than recognizing this is how I should feel, given the situations with which and through which I have lived. I must say with sincere gratitude, that I thank GOD for my loneliness and anxiety, as they really keep me close to AA. When I was a newcomer, I believed in the idea that the meetings were the only antidotes to those feelings and, for the most part, I have found this to be true.

My children are now grown, educated, and solvent. I see cracks in their apparently successful lives, and it is a struggle for me not to take responsibility for their faults, but I believe they have a God watching over them. My half-brothers are steeped in alcoholism. One of them makes sexual advances to my nieces and my daughter, and physically attacked me at a family picnic this summer. My expectations that my family will be happily reunited have been blown all to hell. It is excruciatingly painful for me to be around them or their families for more than ten minutes.

I see most of my 25+ years of recovery has been to a large degree, playing out my earliest beginnings. Relationships of all kinds have been very painful and hard to sustain because—up to this point-I have picked emotionally unavailable, passive/aggressive men, and critical men and women who betray confidences. Trust has been a huge issue for me. I have a small knot of true friends from adolescence and some from AA, but I find life to be rather lonely perhaps because again, my expectations of recovery are such that I think I should have many, many friends. I am not comfortable in large social gatherings. I become emotionally drained around people. My batteries are recharged by being alone and creating things of value to me—a slipcover, or developing a customer base on my laptop.

The three most important elements of staying sober for me are—despite my doubts—asking God to keep me sober every day; attending meetings of all kinds; sharing in the commitment to sponsorship; and, clearing away the carnage of my alcoholism via the 12 steps of AA.

Case Study:
Pamela's Story

"The Booze Made It All OK"

I never felt at home on this planet. Maybe I was from Mars, anywhere, but not from here. I felt this way about my parents as well. Who were these people? They said they were my parents, but I didn't feel connected to them. As a matter of fact, I felt disconnected from the whole human race. I used to study people—how they laughed, what made them cry, what it was that made them happy—all so that I could mimic them. I learned to be a chameleon … and a fraud.

Happiness was the one thing that always eluded me. I would observe people being happy and enjoying their life and I'd think to myself, "When are they going to wake up and face reality?" My reality was pain and loss and sorrow. How could it be possible for someone to have a reality of happiness and peace? I felt that when the "Book of Life" was handed out in Heaven, it never reached me, and I couldn't let anyone know that I didn't know how to live. So I drank. When I drank I didn't care that I was from Mars, living with a bunch of strangers, and it didn't matter that I didn't get that Rule Book for living. The booze made it all OK and I can honestly say now, with almost eight years of being clean and sober, that without booze I never would have lived long enough to get to Alcoholics Anonymous. That feeling of rightness with the world that booze provided kept me from killing myself.

I came from a violent, alcoholic home that appeared middle-class, suburban, and normal. The need to maintain this "illusion" was so great that my parents' reaction to my three nervous breakdowns by the age of nineteen was, "You are not going to some hospital where you'll talk about us and blame us for all your troubles, and besides, what would the neighbors think?" I've often wondered, what did the neighbors think?

The last few years of my parents' drinking dissolved into a fury of screaming rages, violence, broken furniture, bones, and hearts. My mother never dressed, then never bathed, then never lived through it. I was forced to leave home when I was fourteen after being beaten so badly that I knew in my heart if I were to stay I would appear on the front page of the Daily News as another fatality of domestic violence. I lived in a hotel. I tried going home from time to time but it only got worse (it always does when it's alcoholism).

My parents died of the disease and I pretended to mourn them but what I really felt was relief. I felt I was evil for feeling that, and it wasn't until I was sober for many years that I admitted it and began to heal. I realized that it was normal to feel relief. I had been living in a life-threatening madhouse. The parents that I loved had died long before the disease killed their bodies. I drank through their death—through all my feelings of guilt—and used their death as a license to do what ever I pleased. What I wanted to do was drink, drug, sleep-around, and not take any responsibility for any of it. If someone didn't like it, I would show them the door. The door opened and closed many, many times until finally it closed and stayed closed. I had drunk away everything I ever loved, everyone that ever cared about me, and almost, almost drank away my very soul.

I believe that when we are born, there is within us a great light and that when we fulfill our destiny here, this light becomes so brilliant that it shines right through our skin. Alcoholism and the dark places where it led me almost put out my light forever. I could feel the feeble flame flickering and I knew that even though I was only 28 years old, this was my last chance, and that the drink in my hand was my last drink. This precious moment was transformed into a gift of sobriety, and it shines like a beacon of courage—the courage to change, to let go, to grow up and to take responsibility. It powers the courage to bring up all those feelings that were pushed down for so many years, and to continue to uncover, discover, and discard, to keep the best of who I am and deal with the worst. I can say I love you today because I love me. We are all on a journey guarding our light and the light is love, forgiveness, and healing. It is said that if you can survive that which can kill you it will make you strong and happy and free. Surely A.A. has given me this.

An important component to long term recovery for those who were raised in an alcoholic/troubled home is to explore the wounds suffered during childhood. Low self-esteem, co-dependency, shame, and guilt are often deeply implanted in the individual from such an environment. John Bradshaw, author and PBS-TV host explains, "In every case we developed a dependency on things outside ourselves to the point of self-neglect. We gave up our own reality to take care of our parent (s) or the needs of the family system. In short, we survived by having our true self abandoned. We survived by not being there. Co-dependence is the loss of one's inner reality and an addiction to our outer reality."[142]

In the book, *The Psychodynamics of Family Life*, author N. Ackerman states that many mental illnesses develop within a dysfunctional family system. He concludes, "The image of self and the image of the family are reciprocally interdependent."[143]

In Mary-Ellen's story we see a child born into an alcoholic home where chaotically mixed messages discolor her self-esteem and lead her down the same path of destructive drinking. Now with over 40 years of continuous sobriety we can learn by her example that sobriety is not a perfect life where nothing bad or challenging ever happens. In fact it is life on life's terms. Facing and accepting the reality of one's life with responsibility and faith is a major tenet in maintaining sobriety.

Case Study:
Mary Ellen's Story

"The Invisible Line"

I was born in Los Angeles, California. My mother was from New Jersey and my father from Colombia, South America. My mother was 25 years younger than my father and I sensed that he was very jealous of her, especially as she became more "worldly". Both were party people. My mother drank until she was 92, although she would drink only champagne in her later years. My father was an alcoholic. Once he started, he would drink for several days until he had to get a shot from his doctor. He was a periodic drunk, and I remember he told me on a January day, "Don't worry, I will not drink until October." and I noticed that he made good on that statement. My father had a wonderful personality. He worked as a promoter, and he was so well-connected and resourceful, that he could get anything his clients and others needed and wanted. After celebrating a business deal at the Waldorf Astoria in New York City during the World War II, he went to bed and died in his sleep. He was 58.

As for me, I was very shy child, and awkward, though bold enough to be naughty at times. I felt my mother put me down and scolded me too often, so I felt resentment towards her for most of my life. It seemed to me that my mother never had time for me or my sister, who is five years younger than I. We always had what she called "nurses" while growing up. I hated them all, and this is why I believe I ended up being rebellious during my teenage years.

Our family traveled a lot back and forth between the Colombia and the United States while my father was alive. I therefore attended many schools in both countries. I recall that I loved the schools in the United States, but thought the ones in Columbia were too religious.

I had my first drink when I was fourteen. I wanted to see what it was all about, because there was always a lot of drinking and a house was full of people when I was a child. I always said to myself, though, that I was never going to drink, and I did not for two years after that first taste. At sixteen, though, I went to a party, where I felt very shy and afraid to dance. Then, someone handed me a rum & coke, and my whole world changed. From then on I used alcohol to make me feel like "other people"—with no fear, no shyness, and feeling at ease and not at dis-ease. I was not a daily drinker because I did not want to continually have hangovers—in fact, only once in 25 years of drinking did I drink daily, and that was over a 3-day stretch. During the last 15 years of my drinking, I regularly mixed alcohol and tranquilizers.

As the years went by, my drinking—but most of all the feelings of guilt—got worse, and as I look back on the summer of 1952, I crossed the "invisible" line, meaning I underwent a personality change. I became aggressive and started to loose my inhibitions and to be "free". I experienced blackouts from the beginning, but was never arrested for driving under the influence, nor was I ever hospitalized for intoxication. I found that during my alcoholic years, I did not lose "things", but I did lose friends, as well as a husband, who also drank.

I moved, with my nine-year-old son, and a nanny, from Columbia to New York, because I thought that, in the city, no one would "bug" me. My son, it occurs to me as I write this, has been sober for the past nine years with AA.

I drank for 25 years and hit bottom December, 1964 on Christmas Eve. For a month after that, things got worse, and in January, of 1965, I told an AA member that I was a "potential" alcoholic and I attended an AA meeting.

I use the AA program to stay sober, to take one day at a time, and to follow the Twelve Steps. I also go to meetings to help people, and I have changed my way of thinking. Though my use of the tools stays the same, I sometimes use the program more often than at other times. My sobriety date is January 14, 1965 and I have been sober ever since. I was on tranquilizers for many years and I am aware that I have an addictive personality. For the last year I have had anxiety and perhaps depression due to emphysema, heart problems—chronic obstructive pulmonary disease—and I am having trouble adjusting to my health problems. The AA program and a few people help me with this.

I have forty years of sobriety and I use the basic tools of AA—my Six Spiritual Beliefs are more than religious, and I have also been going to Catholic Mass every Sunday for the last three years. I try to exercise (I used to play tennis and golf) but with my breathing problems, this can be difficult to do. I try to pray and or meditate, and I go to one or two AA meetings a week. I also take courses at the Museum and perform service work for others in AA. The most important elements to maintaining my sobriety are: God as I understand Him, living in the present, and loving while trying not to feel negative emotions.

12

ENDURING SOBRIETY

As a result of my research study and my professional and personal experience over the past 26+ years in the area of addiction and 12-step programs, I have developed a treatment program that is holistic in nature but holographic in form. One of the unique characteristics of a hologram is that each of its parts has the ability to re-create the whole. I remember as a child being fascinated by starfish. If any one of the starfish legs were cut off, the fish had the ability to grow another one and survive. As alcoholics and addicts in recovery, perhaps a similar ability is needed to sustain long term abstinence and well being.

The issue of "reproductive transcendence" or "spiritual adaptability" are integral to this treatment model. Take for example the feeling of rebirth that often accompanies the "pink cloud" of early sobriety. The newly sober person feels elation at not only being free from the bondage of compulsive drinking, but also at the promise of a new and better life sober. In my experience this is not a solitary event experienced only by the newly sober. It is a living process, as is spiritual and emotional growth, a process that continues to recreate, renew, and redefine itself as it exists in any given moment. I am not the person I was last year, nor will I be the same next year or the year after.

'One Day at a Time' in Holographic Treatment

How I choose to grow and manifest, whether it be positive or negative, loving or fearful, sober or drunk is a daily choice. The premise of living one day at a time is very pertinent in approaching this transformational treatment model. The concept of living one day at a time was adopted by Alcoholics Anonymous from the spiritual teachings of Mathew Fox. The message is a literal one—even though it is more often than not interpreted subjectively. If we live in today, for it is the only time we truly have, and it is always today—then the message is clear. The focus of time is then relegated to the "now". How then do we practice living in the now when there are things in the past that are unresolved, and, as such, discolor our perception of the both the present and the future?

Chuck C. was a sober member of Alcoholics Anonymous for over 40 years before he passed away. Chuck had a very powerful message, and became as a result a circuit speaker in A.A. I had the opportunity on several occasions in the late 1970's to hear him speak. His message was clear, "Uncover the pain from the past, Discover how it is impacting the present and Discard that which is not helpful to sobriety and good living." I have paraphrased his message but the content is the basis of my treatment model, along with steps 4–10 in the 12 steps for healing the wounds and wreckage of the individual's past. Journaling, telling one's story, sharing secrets and shameful behavior, owning our part in the destruction of relationships, jobs and self-esteem, changing destructive and/or self centered/self-seeking behaviors, holding oneself fully accountable for everything that is in one's life. It is not with shame and guilt, but rather with compassion and understanding that we form a loving relationship with the inner child, and thus allow him or her to heal. In this way, one can emerge from the frozen state entered as a result of early trauma, and integrate the child into the adult's consciousness. These are some of the tools and commitments necessary to freeing oneself from the negative effects of the past and the wounded subconscious mind. It has been my experience as a therapist that if this is not done, the past and its wounds act almost like a ball and chain keeping the individual stuck in the very pain he or she wants so desperately to escape.

The Works of Grof and Peck in Developing Holographic Treatment

The human condition is subject to the laws of the linear world. The time/space continuum is dictated by the laws of cause and effect. The seeds I plant, the actions I take, the words I speak, and the beliefs I nurture all make themselves manifest in time. Taking a very conscious approach to this creative law can turn the tide in one's favor. This law of cause and effect is true not just on the emotional and physical plane; but on the spiritual plane as well. In the East, it is called karma, and the West defines it as Judgment Day. Whatever concept is used, the premise is to heal, learn, and create within conscious, subconscious, and "super-conscious" states of reality. What exactly is a super-conscious state of reality? I have developed this perspective in part through a study of the groundbreaking work of Dr. Stanislav Grof over the last twenty years. Grof's holotropic research into non-ordinary states of consciousness has opened the way for other transpersonal theorists.

Holotropic, as defined by Dr.Stanislav Grof is the state of "whole learning" or 'turning towards wholeness".[144] Grof's work centers around psychotherapeutic techniques that allow clients to heal, not just emotionally and physically, but deeply within their souls as well. Holotropic states encourage the individual to heal on all levels of consciousness. They encourage spiritual transcendence, personality transformation and the evolution of the individual's consciousness.[145]

Grof has an expanding view of the human potential and feels that Western Academic science is limited in its perception of human consciousness. He proposes that "materialistic science has an incomplete and inadequate model of reality ... the nature of consciousness and the relationship between consciousness and matter, particularly in the brain, have to be radically revised." His belief is that in the not-too-distant future, "transpersonal psychology and work with nonordinary states of consciousness will become the new science paradigm."[146] Super consciousness, then, is a heightened state of awareness encompassing all four dimensions (possibly more) in which the observer relates to himself/herself primarily as a spiritual being existing temporarily in a physical reality for the purpose of learning and service. So like the transpersonal work of Dr. Grof, the self of the ego and personality is then "freed" to become an expanded "Self". But how is this achieved, and is it available to everyone? I offer as a blueprint the principles set forth in my Holographic Treatment Model. Scott Peck, in his book, *The Road Less Traveled and Beyond*, describes his theory on the stages of spiritual growth as follows:

Stage 1:   Anti-Social, superficial "belief system" with no basic principals.

Stage 2:   Formal institutional/formal religion and practice.

Stage 3:   Skeptic/scientific-minded, rational, interested in what can be "proven".

Stage 4:   Mystical/Communal—Feeling deeply connected to a "Higher Power" and comfortable with the mystery of all that is sacred. [147]

Stage 4 seems to align itself with the experiences people have in the 12 step program. The feeling of being a part of something greater than yourself and yet being a very important contributor to the community's overall existence. Feelings of usefulness help to heal low self esteem and feelings of guilt and shame. Helping others to achieve sobriety by sharing one's experiences has a profoundly healing and unifying effect on both the giver and the receiver.

The Holographic Treatment Plan

Holographic super-consciousness uses the 12 steps of Alcoholics Anonymous, the four stages of Peck's spiritual growth model, and Grof's transpersonal holotropic treatment model as springboards to a new theory "beyond the 12 steps".

Phase One (The Foundation)

- Achieve sobriety and continue, as a life style, practicing the steps and princi-pals of the A.A. program. This includes: regular, weekly attendance at meet-ings (other 12-step programs may also be added), working the steps and the process of developing character and accountability with a sponsor who is an active, sober member of A.A.; being of service to the program as a whole and the "home" group in particular which includes sponsoring and assisting other alcoholics; regularly speaking and sharing at meetings, one on one, and at con-ventions.

- Continue to read and study spiritual material and practice conscious contact with your Higher Power through the disciplines of prayer and meditation.

- Aid the physical body to facilitate the effects of active alcoholism by eating a healthy variety of whole foods and when necessary following a hypoglycemic diet if low blood sugar is an issue(this is the case with many alcoholics as is the issue of an over production of yeast).

- Exercise daily, rekindling a relationship with your natural surroundings, culti-vating benefits of good grooming and self care.

- Develop a healthy mental diet. What we think and the things we affirm are just as crucial to our well being as the foods we eat. It may be true that you are what you eat, but it is equally true that you are what you think and you create what you believe to be true.

- Stop creating with your thoughts and unconscious affirmations what you fear and start creating what they truly want. Think before you speak. Make sure what you put the "I am" to is what you really want to be identified with, for example: 'I am so fat and no matter I do I can't loose weight' hinges on the limitation of "Can't", which is a powerless, responsibility-lacking word. It is best not to use it unless that is what you truly want. When I say truly want—I mean not what one may "feel" is true but what you wish to be true in you heart. So instead of saying the above negative affirmation and planting seeds for a limiting self-fulfilling prophecy, adjust the observation to be that of a gentle observer, one that is compassionate and helpful—"I have extra weight on my body that is not helpful to my health and well being. Just for today I make a commitment to myself to eat only the foods that are most helpful for my body's performance and vitality". The second and most important part is to then throughout the day consciously ask yourself before eating anything, "Is this helpful to my well being?" If the answer is 'no'—do not do it—just for today.

- Eliminate guilt. It is a learned emotion and it can be unlearned. In the immortal words of Jiminy Cricket, "Let your conscious be your guide." We know when something is not right for us. We feel it in our gut. Follow that awareness and there will be no need for guilt.

- Explore tools to aid in the transformation of your thinking from primarily negative to positive and optimistic. Daily affirmations, creative visualization, biofeedback, daily positive reading of spiritual materials etc. can be very helpful. We live in a dualistic existence—the world of opposites: good/bad; right/wrong; healthy/sick. We have a choice between optimistic and pessimistic. Why would you choose the latter? Start choosing the positive, even if it doesn't feel quite real at first. If you practice this choice just for "today", positive outcomes will manifest themselves in your life. Just remember, many of us have been affirming the negative for decades, so, as you begin shifting your perception, give it time.

- Heal and deal with the past: its wounds, traumas, the effects of your "inner child". Uncover core beliefs, self-defeating patterns of behavior and negative self-image and/or loathing.

- Develop a loving relationship with your inner child—transform the child from wounded to magical and creative.

- Identify and heal all fragmented aspects of yourself, and integrate these parts into a strong self image. As the saying goes: "If you know who you are, no one else can name you."

- Learn the art of self evaluation. Drop guilt and extreme images of oneself and become "right sized". Learn how to determine what is the best choice for yourself based on understanding your strengths and weaknesses, and the goals you are aspiring to fulfill.

- Develop and maintain healthy relationships at home, in the workplace, and in your community. Heal your co-dependency issues, which can include rescuing, people-pleasing and chameleon-like personality shifts (the fraud), and any roles developed out of a dysfunctional (ACoA) family of origin.

- Discover and remove any obstacles to your health and happiness.

- Discover your talents and gifts and uncover work that is important for you to do based on these assets.

- Practice honesty, love and service in all areas of your life.

- Practice silence and introspection. Align with that which is "right" for you and hold to it.

- Learn time management techniques, goal setting/fulfilling, and each year take the time and effort to create both one—and five-year plans (which would include emotional, physical, financial, spiritual and mental goals). For example: Plan to be more thoughtful, to refrain from gossiping, or to set aside more time for prayer and meditation. After the goals are clear, set a strategy for implementation with a timeline. Follow and chart your progress through the plan.

- Create balance in all areas, following the whole concept of "Being" and "Doing". Shift away from the concept of a "human being" or a "human doing" to a continual state of a "human becoming".

- Practice and affirm gratitude for all the gifts in one's life.

Phase Two: The Transformation

- Examine and continue to strengthen the tools and rewards of phase one: healing childhood wounds, loving relationships in life/work/community, authentic self development-an authentic self is honest in word and deed and operates out of a sense of personal rightness and commitment, and self-esteem.

The authentic and empowered being is now ready for another metamorphosis—an internal exploration beyond the perimeters of the three dimensional world. Many have already had a glimpse of this world through the regular practice of prayer and meditation and yogic postures. The ego/personality self that is now healthy and happy can let go into a transpersonal identity that emerges as a spiritual Self, co-creating with God. For some the co-creating will take on very lofty proportions and for others it will be a quiet, internal change that only the individual will experience. The outer world of this person appears to be the same. So what is the difference and how does one begin the journey? The third step in the 12 step program is the starting point and the enormity of the decision is taken piecemeal as the person grows and heals. Many years—perhaps a whole life-time—will be necessary to totally comprehend the implications and the challenges of practicing the 3rd step absolutely. It reads, "Made a decision to turn our will and our life over to the care of God." It might be helpful to take this step apart to ponder its true connotation. 'Made' implies created by means of a decision (a focus and intention) to turn (or give fully and absolutely the only gift we truly have—which is our free will). God gave us free will. By giving our free will back to His care, we have made a complete journey. God gave us the freedom to live and operate our will without interference. Whatever we created—good or bad—from that gift was our right. By surrendering our will and our lives over to the care of God we are surrendering the limited will of the ego to the immortal and limitless Will of God. The Will of God is only good, loving, and abundant. We are in fact committing to co-create with the power of the universe instead of aligning with the petty hopes and fears of a mortal ego. We can continue to love and appreciate the human existence but we nurture and feed primarily our soul and the souls of our fellows. We strive to achieve this by:

- Regularly going on spiritual retreats and solitary retreats.

- Continuing to deepen meditation and yoga practice to keep the physical body/mind open and receptive to higher levels of consciousness.

- Practicing anonymous giving and service to others.

- Making all decisions based on love and not on fear.

- Developing through a lifetime of practice, trust in the Will of God.

Phase Three: The Super-Consciousness State

- Continue to take spiritual inventory uncovering any thoughts of lack, limitation, doubt, or hate (including self-hate).

- Become an unencumbered creative living force for good and love in the world.

- Love God more than you love your ego identity.

- Practicing conscious living and strategies for conscious dying.

- Continue to seek out mentors and teachers in all the above practices. Give away what you have in order to keep it.

- Practice detachment by recognizing the temporal nature of this existence. Detachment is not lack of feeling, it is lack of ownership and control.

- Live and give as if it were your last day on earth and plan as if you will live forever.

- Discover your purpose and fulfill it to the best of your ability—no matter what the cost.

- Discover your truth and speak to anyone who will listen—no matter what the cost.

- Acknowledge that all experience has been helpful to personal growth and compassion. Forgiveness is a natural extension of this mindset.

- Practice giving unmerited gifts.

- Be authentic—no matter what the cost.

- Live an extraordinary life—no matter what the cost.

- Learn to love completely and absolutely—no matter what the cost.

Having briefly outlined the Holographic Treatment Model, we find a model not just for recovering alcoholics and addicts, but for any human being choosing the path of transformation. The recovering alcoholic has, ironically, an advantage over the "normal" folk in that they practice the 12 steps and the principals of the program in order to not pick up a drink. The search for God and the development of a healthy spiritual condition is tantamount for enduring sobriety. The addict becomes spiritually aligned in order to stay alive—there is no wiggle room if he or she wants to get better. So what starts out as a "fait accompli" for the alcoholic becomes in fact the gateway to a life of miraculous change and transformation—a life that is, as many alcoholics in recovery affirm—second to none.

This research project was perhaps most illuminating by what was not said in all these stories and interviews and yet was a thread that was woven throughout each individual's sobriety. What enabled them to endure the pain and hardships of active alcoholism and early recovery to go on to achieve an enduring sobriety for over twenty years? Perhaps it was the realization that when they stood before their God, having hit a demoralizing bottom from addiction, at their worst, surrounded by countless bad deeds, selfishness, self-centeredness and darkness, that God smiled and blessed them with the gift of sobriety. It is in the healing power of an unmerited gift that unconditional love is truly experienced, and, once felt, heals everything around it instantly and forever more.

Endnotes

[1]. Schaef, A. (1987). *When society becomes an addict.* Cambridge: Harper & Row.

[2]. Kennedy, L. (2005, February 17) Medications help alcoholics control drinking. *Behavioral Health News Service.* Retrieved April 9, 2005 from http://www.hbns.org/news/drinking 02–17–05.cfm

[3]. Nester, E. & Malenka, R. (2004, March). The addicted brain. *Scientific American*, p. 85.

[4]. Milam, J. R., Ketcham, K. (1983). *Under the Influence: A guide to the myths and realities of alcoholism.* New York: Bantam. p. 8

[5]. Milam & Ketcham, p. 83

[6]. Scheaf, p.32

[7]. Pert, p.24

[8]. Pert, p.22

[9]. Kennedy, para. 9

[10]. Milam & Ketcham 25

[11]. Milam & Ketcham 27

[12]. Milam & Ketcham 31

[13]. Milam & Ketcham 17

[14]. Milam & Ketcham 18

[15]. Milam & Ketcham 18

[16]. Milam & Ketcham 18

[17]. Milam & Ketcham 19

[18].   Hamburg, M. (1986, August). The nature of craving. *Vogue*, p. 322

[19].   Hamburg 332–333

[20].   Gordis, Enoch. (1996, July). Alcohol-Alert, Neuroscience Research and Medications Development. *National Institute on Alcohol Abuse and Alcoholism*, p. 3

[21].   Gordis 5–6

[22].   Gordis 7–8

[23].   Ibid, pp. 9–11

[24].   McGowan, K. (2004, Nov/Dec). Pay Attention to This!, (Nora Volkow) [Interview]. *Psychology Today, 37*(6), p. 88.

[25].   Gordis, p. 88

[26].   McGowan, p. 89

[27].   Ibid, p. 90

[28].   Ibid, p. 89

[29].   Alcohol, violence, & aggression. (1997, October). *National Institute on Alcohol Abuse and Alcoholism.* (NIAAA)Alcohol Alert: No. 38. Paragraph 18

[30].   Gibbons, p.21

[31].   Alcohol Abuse Increases, dependence declines across decade: Young adult minorities emerge as high-risk subgroups. (2004, June 10). *National Institutes of Health (NIH) News*

[32].   Gibbons 27

[33].   Gibbons 27

[34].   Gibbons 21

[35].   Milam & Ketcham, pp. 43–45

[36].   Gibbons, p. 28

[37].   Milam & Ketcham, p. 43

[38]. Merton, R. K. and. Nesbet, R. A. (1966). *Contemporary Social Problems.* New York: Harcourt

[39]. McCarthy, R. G. & Douglass, E. M. (1949). *Alcohol and Social Responsibility: A New Educational Approach.* New York: Crowell

[40]. Slack, D. (2004, March 14) Drinking games: Boston Uncommon, *The Boston Globe Magazine*, p.9

[41]. Robertson, Nan. (1992, February-March). Addiction and aging. *Modern Maturity*, p. 41.

[42]. Substance Abuse Among Women in the US, Substance Abuse and Mental Health Services Administration (SAMHSA) Dept. of Health and Human Services, 1996

[43]. Jacob, T. and Leonard K. (1994). *Family and peer influences in the development of adolescent alcohol abuse."* National Inst. On Alcohol Abuse and Alcoholism, Research Monograph # 26 (Bethesda, MD,

[44]. Milam & Ketcham, p. 31

[45]. Milam & Ketcham, p. 83

[46]. Milam & Ketcham, p. 83

[47]. Gibbons, p. 14

[48]. Milam & Ketcham, p. 81

[49]. Freud, Sigmund. *Five lectures on psycho-analysis.* Strachey, J. (Ed. & Trans.) (1977). New York: Norton, p. 275

[50]. DiChiara, G., Acquas, E. and Tanda, G. (1996) Ethanol is a neurochemical surrogate of conventional reinforcers. *Alcohol, 13*, p. 23

[51]. Milam & Ketcham, p. 34

[52]. Goodwin, D.W. (1978). The genetics of alcoholism: A state of the art review. *Alcohol Health & Research World* 2(3), p. 9

[53]. Blakeslee, Sandra. (1984, 14 August) Scientists find key biological cause of alcoholism. *New York Times.* p. C1.

[54]. Blakesee, p. C1

[55]. Bloom, Floyd, et al, eds. (1982) Beta-carbolines and tetrahydroiso-quinolines. Proceedings of a Salk Institute workshop held in La Jolla, CA December, 1981. *Progress in Clinical and Biological Research (90)*. New York: Liss

[56]. Blakesee, p. C1

[57]. Schuckit, M., & Rayses, V. (1979). Ethanol ingestion: Differences in blood acetaldehyde concentrations in relatives of alcoholics and controls. *Science, 203*, p. 54

[58]. Davis B.E. & Walsh M.J. (1970) Alcohol, amines and alkaloids: A possible biochemical basis for alcohol addiction. *Science, 167*, pp. 1005–1007.

[59]. Hamburg, p. 333

[60]. Hamburg, p. 333

[61]. Milam & Ketcham, p. 83

[62]. Bodian, S. (1988, November/December) Dealing with our addictions: The connection between spirituality and addictive behavior. *Yoga Journal*. p.40

[63]. Bodian, S. (1988, November/December) Addiction to Perfection: An interview with Marion Woodman, *Yoga Journal*. p.52

[64]. Dardis, T. (1989). *The thirsty muse, alcohol and the American writer*. New York: Ticknor & Fields, p. 133

[65]. Milam & Ketcham, p. 59

[66]. Dardis, p.132

[67]. Milam & Ketcham, p. 64

[68]. Dardis, p.252

[69]. Gorham, C. O. (1958) *Wine of life: A novel about Balzac*. New York: Dial Press, p.328

[70]. Fitzgerald, F. S. (1969). *The last tycoon : an unfinished novel* New York : Scribner's, p. 97

[71]. Milam & Ketcham, p. 83

[72]. Palmer, Louise Danielle. (2005, September-October) The next gender revolution. *Spirituality and Health*, p. 30

[73]. Ibid, p. 34

[74].) Alcohol Alert #10: Alcohol and Women, (1994) National Institutes on Alcohol Abuse and Alcoholism (NIAAA).

[75]. Palmer 34

[76]. Gibbons 37

[77]. Baekeland, Frederick. (1977) Evaluation of Treatment Methods in Chronic Alcoholism. *Treatment and Rehabilitation of the Chronic Alcoholic*, B. Kissen and H. Begleiter, eds., p. 389. New York: Plenum Press.

[78]. Gibbons 19

[79]. Ibid

[80]. Chastain 39

[81]. Dupree, L.W.; Broskowski, H.; and Schonfeld, L. (1984) The Gerontology Alcohol Project: A behavioral treatment program for elderly alcohol abusers. *Gerontologist* 24, p. 511,

[82]. UPI/CBS News, St Louis, 9/3/2004

[83]. Jung, C. G. (1933) *Modern man in search of a soul* (Del, W. S. & Baynes, C. F., Trans.)

New York : Harcourt. p.229

[84]. Wilson, W. G. (1958, April 28). *Alcoholics Anonymous—Beginning and Growth*. Speech to the New York Medical Society on Alcoholism

[85]. Wilson, 1958

[86]. Milam & Ketcham 142–3

[87]. Peck M. S. (1993). *Further Along the Road Less Traveled: The unending journey toward spiritual growth.* New York: Simon & Schuster. [Excerpt: *New Age Journal* (1993, Nov./Dec.) p. 54

[88]. NIAAA, No. 38, 1997

[89]. Brown, L. P. (1995, January). The drug problem is everybody's problem. *Hazelden News and Professional Update.* p.3.

[90]. AA survey, 2001

[91]. Milam & Ketcham 31

[92]. Dardis 19

[93]. Wilson, 1946, p. 21

[94]. Wilson, 1946, p. 21

[95]. Luks, A. & Barbato, J. (1989). *You are what you drink: The authoritative report on what alcohol does to the body, mind and longevity.* New York: Villard, p. 36

[96]. Luks & Barbato 36

[97]. Gottlieb, W. (1979, December). Nutrition: The silver lining. *Prevention.* p. 178

[98]. Rogers L. L. & Pelton, R.B. (1957). Glutamine in the treatment of alcoholism, A preliminary report. *Quarterly Journal of Studies of Alcoholism, 18*, p. 581.

[99]. Rogers & Pelton 581

[100]. Underwood, A. & Adler, J. (2005, January 17). Diet and Genes. *Newsweek, 145*(3). p. 41

[101]. Underwood 43

[102]. Bruce, J. (1991, September/October). Twelve-Step Research: Trying to Measure the Immeasurable. *Common Boundary.* p. 34

[103]. Bruce 34

[104]. Bruce 35

[105]. Bruce 34

[106]. Nester, E. & Malenka, R. (2004, March). The addicted brain. *Scientific American*, p. 85.

[107]. Harwood, H. Fountain, D.; and Livermore, G. (1998) Updating Estimates of the economic costs of alcohol abuse in the United States: Estimates. *National Institute on Alcohol Abuse and Alcoholism (NIAA)*.

[108]. Kennedy 1

[109]. Toft, Doug. (1995, January) The Minnesota Model: Humane, Holistic, Flexible. *Hazelden News & Professional Update.* p. 2

[110]. Toft 1

[111]. Toft 2

[112]. Reyes, K. W. (1992, February-March), There is so much help out there." (Betty Ford) [Interview]. *Modern Maturity.* p. 29

[113]. Vacovsky, L. Finding effective treatment for alcohol dependence. *American Council on Alcoholism.* Retrieved 5/16/05, from: http://www.aca-usa.org/pharm2.htm

[114]. Maricq HR, Jarvik LF, Rainer JD. (1969 Nov 8) Schizophrenia and depression of lymphocyte response to P.H.A. *Lancet.* 2(7628). p. 1011

[115]. Gordis, para. 4

[116]. Rawson R., McCann, M., Hasson, A. (2000) Pharmacotherapies for substance abuse treatment: The beginning of a new era. Counselor, Retrieved April 29, 2005 from http://www.counselor magazine.com/display_article.asp?aid= Pharmacotherapies_for_Substance_Abuse_Treatment.asp

[117]. Kennedy para. 6

[118]. Kennedy para. 4

[119]. Kennedy para. 9

[120]. Menzies, P. Why is recovery from Alcoholism so difficult? And is there hope for successful treatment? *American Council on Alcoholism*. Retrieved May 16, 2005, from: http://www.aca–usa.org/pharm2.htm. para 16

[121]. Rawson para 4

[122]. Rawson para 4

[123]. Banaszynski, Jacqui. (1992, February/March). Ties that blind: Facing up to the family secret. *Modern Maturity*. p. 64

[124]. Stone, D. The royal road to recovery. (1988, Nov/Dec.) *Yoga Journal*, p. 87

[125]. Williams, C. & Laird, R. (1992, Sept/Oct.) Beyond A.A. *New Age Journal*, p. 38.

[126]. Chalfin, Barry. (1999, Fall) Addiction: Is it Starting To Overshadow Your Life? *Many Hands*, p. 15

[127]. Chalfin 23

[128]. *Alcoholics Anonymous* (1977). 3rd Edition. New York: General Services Office, PP. 59–60

[129]. Wilson. W.G. (1939) *Twelve steps and twelve traditions*. New York: General Services Office, Alcoholics Anonymous, P. 21

[130]. Alcoholic Anonymous, 1977, p. 570

[131]. Alcoholic Anonymous, 1977, p. 63

[132]. Sikorsky I.I. Jr. (1990) *A.A.'s Godparents: Three early influences on Alcoholics Anonymous and its foundation*. Minneapolis: Compcare. pp. 47–48

[133]. Alcoholic Anonymous, 1977, pp. 83–84

[134]. Peck [excerpts], 1993, p. 56

[135]. *Alcoholics Anonymous*. (2002). The Serenity Prayer: A brief summary of its origin. New York: General Services Office.

[136]. Sikorsky 3

[137]. Gorski 1993

[138]. Alcoholics Anonymous 1977 p. 33

[139]. Alcoholics Anonymous 1977 p. 23

[140]. Alcoholics Anonymous 1977 p. 569

[141]. Sikorsky 12

[142]. Bodian 45

[143]. Bradshaw, John. (1988). *The family: A revolutionary way to self discovery.* Deerfield Beach, Florida: Health Communications. p. 23.

[144]. Grof M.D.,Stanislav. (2004, June/August). Mind and healing: Psychology of the future." *Shift Magazine.*, p. 20.

[145]. Grof 22

[146]. Grof 22

[147]. Peck M. S. (1997) *The road less traveled & beyond: Spiritual growth in an age of anxiety.* New York: Simon & Schuster. p. 247

References

Addiction, (1999, Mar). Interview with LeClair Bissell; 94(3), 321–327

Alcoholics Anonymous (1977). 3rd Edition. New York: General Services Office

Alcoholics Anonymous. (2002). The Serenity Prayer: A brief summary of its origin. New York: General Services Office.

Baekeland, Frederick. (1977). Evaluation of Treatment Methods in Chronic Alcoholism. *Treatment and Rehabilitation of the Chronic Alcoholic*, B. Kissen and H. Begleiter, eds., pp. 385—440. New York: Plenum Press,

Banaszynski, Jacqui. (1992, February/March). Ties that blind: Facing up to the family secret. *Modern Maturity.*

Becker, H. S. (1986). *Writing for social scientists: How to start and finish your thesis, book, or article.* University of Chicago Press.

Blakeslee, Sandra. (1984, 14 August) Scientists find key biological cause of alcoholism. *New York Times.* p. C1.

Bloom, Floyd, et al, eds. (1982) Beta-carbolines and tetrahydroisoquinolines. Proceedings of a Salk Institute workshop held in La Jolla, CA December, 1981. *Progress in Clinical and Biological Research (90).* New York: Liss

Bodian, S. (1988, November/December) Dealing with our addictions: The connection between spirituality and addictive behavior. pp. 38–45. Addiction to Perfection: An interview with Marion Woodman, p.52 *Yoga Journal.*

Bradshaw, John. (1988). *The family: A revolutionary way to self discovery.* Deerfield Beach, Florida: Health Communications.

Brown, L. P. (1995, January). The drug problem is everybody's problem. *Hazelden News and Professonal Update.*

Bruce, J. (1991, September/October). Twelve-Step Research: Trying to Measure the Immeasurable. *Common Boundary.*

Chalfin, Barry. (1999, Fall) Addiction: Is it Starting To Overshadow Your Life? *Many Hands*, 13–18

Chastain, S. (1992, February-March). The accidental addict, *Modern Maturity*. 38–49

Crittenden, Jules. (2005, March 7). (With Playboy Image, N. Korea's Kim a strong, shrewd leader. *The Boston Herald*, p.10.

Davis B.E. & Walsh M.J. (1970) Alcohol, amines and alkaloids: A possible biochemical basis for alcohol addiction. *Science, 167,* 1005–1007.

Dardis, T. (1989). *The thirsty muse, alcohol and the American writer.* New York: Ticknor &

DiChiara, G., Acquas, E. and Tanda, G. (1996) Ethanol is a neurochemical surrogate of conventional reinforcers. *Alcohol, 13*, 13—17

Dupree, L.W.; Broskowski, H.; and Schonfeld, L. (1984) The Gerontology Alcohol Project: A behavioral treatment program for elderly alcohol abusers. *Gerontologist* 24:510–516

Fitzgerald, F. S. (1969). *The last tycoon : an unfinished novel* New York : Scribner's.

Freud, Sigmund. *Five lectures on psycho-analysis.* Strachey, J. (Ed. & Trans.) (1977). New York: Norton

Gibbons, B. (1992, February). Alcohol, the legal drug. *National Geographic*, *181*(2), 3–35.

Goodwin, D.W. (1978). The genetics of alcoholism: A state of the art review. *Alcohol Health & Research World* 2(3):2–12

Gordis, Enoch. (1996, July). Alcohol-Alert, Neuroscience Research and Medications Development. *National Institute on Alcohol Abuse and Alcoholism*, Publication #33-PH366.

Gorham, C. O. (1958) *Wine of life: A novel about Balzac.* New York: Dial Press

Gorski, T. et al. (1983). Relapse Warning Sign Assessment Form. Hazel Crest, Ill: Herald House Independence Press, re-published as *Relapse prevention and the substance-abusing criminal offender : An executive briefing.* Rockville, MD: U.S. Dept. of Health and Human Services, Public Health Service, *Substance Abuse and Mental Health Services Administration (SAMHSA).*

Gottlieb, W. (1979, December). Nutrition: The silver lining. *Prevention.*

Grof M.D.,Stanislav. (2004, June/August). Mind and healing: Psychology of the future." *Shift Magazine.*, 20–23.

Hamburg, M. (1986, August). The nature of craving. *Vogue*, 328–337

Hart, A. (1990). *Healing Life's Hidden Addictions.* Grand Rapids, MI: Servant

Harwood, H. Fountain, D.; and Livermore, G. (1998) Updating Estimates of the economic costs of alcohol abuse in the United States: Estimates. *National Institute on Alcohol Abuse and Alcoholism (NIAA).* Based on 1992 report by Harwood et al. NIH Publication No. 98–4327. Rockville, MD: *National Institutes of Health,* 1998.

Maricq HR, Jarvik LF, Rainer JD. (1969 Nov 8) Schizophrenia and depression of lymphocyte response to P.H.A. *Lancet.* 2(7628):1008.

Jung, C. G. (1933) *Modern man in search of a soul* (Del, W. S. & Baynes, C. F., Trans.) New York : Harcourt.

Kennedy, L. (2005, February 17) Medications help alcoholics control drinking. *Behavioral Health News Service.* Retrieved April 9, 2005 from http://www.hbns.org/news/drinking02–17–05.cfm

Lofland, J. (1971). *Analyzing social settings: A guide to qualitative observation and analysis.* Belmont, CA: Wadsworth

Luks, A. & Barbato, J. (1989). *You are what you drink: The authoritative report on what alcohol does to the body, mind and longevity.* New York: Villard.

Marrone, R. & Rasor, R. (1972). *Behavior observation and analysis.* San Francisco: Rinehart Press.

McCarthy, R. G. & Douglass, E. M. (1949). *Alcohol and Social Responsibility: A New Educational Approach.* New York: Crowell

McGowan, K. (2004, Nov/Dec). Pay Attention to This!, (Nora Volkow) [Interview]. *Psychology Today, 37*(6), 84–91.

McGue, M. (1997). Genes, Environment and the Etiology of Alcoholism. [Research Monograph # 26] Bethesda, MD: *National Institute on Alcohol Abuse and Alcoholism*

Menzies, P. Why is recovery from Alcoholism so difficult? And is there hope for successful treatment? *American Council on Alcoholism.* Retrieved May 16, 2005, from: http://www.aca-usa.org/pharm2.htm

Merton, R. K. and. Nesbet, R. A. (1966). *Contemporary Social Problems.* New York: Harcourt.

Michaelis, Vicki. (2004, November 9). Swim star Phelps faces DWI charges. *U.S. A. Today,* p. 1C.

Milam, J. R., Ketcham, K. (1983). *Under the Influence: A guide to the myths and realities of alcoholism.* New York: Bantam. p. 8

Alcohol, violence, and aggression. (1997, October). *National Institute on Alcohol Abuse and Alcoholism.* (NIAAA)Alcohol Alert: No. 38.// www.niaaa.nih.gov/publications/aa38.htm. Paragraphs 2, 22

Nester, E. & Malenka, R. (2004, March). The addicted brain. *Scientific American,* p. 85.

Alcohol Abuse Increases, dependence declines across decade: Young adult minorities emerge as high-risk subgroups. (2004, June 10). *National Institutes of Health (NIH) News*

Nester, E. & Malenka, R. (2004, March). The addicted brain. *Scientific American,* 85

Palmer, Louise Danielle. (2005, September-October) The next gender revolution. *Spirituality and Health,* 30–35

Peck M. S. (1993). *Further Along the Road Less Traveled: The unending Journey toward Spiritual Growth.* New York: Simon & Schuster, [Excerpt, *New Age Journal* (1993, Nov./Dec.) p. 54

Peck M. S. (1997) *The road less traveled & beyond: Spiritual growth in an age of anxiety.* New York: Simon & Schuster.

Pert, Candace. (2004, Sept./Nov.). Molecules and choice: Bio-molecular perspective. *Shift Magazine*

Reddy, Betty. (1987). *Alcoholism: A Family Illness.* Park Ridge, Illinois: Parkside Medical Services

Rawson R., McCann, M., Hasson, A. (2000) Pharmacotherapies for substance abuse treatment: The beginning of a new era. Counselor, Retrieved April 29, 2005 from http://www.counselormagazine.com/display_article.asp? aid= Pharmacotherapies_for_Substance_Abuse_Treatment.asp

Reyes, K. W. (1992, February-March), There is so much help out there." (Betty Ford) [Interview]. *Modern Maturity.*

Robertson, Nan. (1992, February-March). Addiction and aging. *Modern Maturity.*

Rogers L. L. & Pelton, R.B. (1957). Glutamine in the treatment of alcoholism, A preliminary report. *Quarterly Journal of Studies of Alcoholism, 18,* 581–587.

Schaef, A. (1987). *When society becomes an addict.* Cambridge: Harper & Row.

Schuckit, M., & Rayses, V. (1979). Ethanol ingestion: Differences in blood acetaldehyde concentrations in relatives of alcoholics and controls. *Science, 203,* 54.

Sikorsky I.I. Jr. (1990) *A.A.'s Godparents: Three early influences on Alcoholics Anonymous and its foundation.* Minneapolis: Compcare.

Slack, D. (2004, March 14) Drinking games: Boston Uncommon, *The Boston Globe Magazine,* p.9

Stone, D. The royal road to recovery. (1988, Nov/Dec.) *Yoga Journal,* 87-.93

Substance Abuse Among Women in the US, Substance Abuse and Mental Health Services Administration (SAMHSA) Dept. of Health and Human Services, 1996. Retrieved May 18, 2005, from: http://www.os.dhhs.gov/news/press/1997pres/970922.html

Toft, Doug. (1995, January) The Minnesota Model: Humane, Holistic, Flexible. *Hazelden News & Professional Update.*

Underwood, A. & Adler, J. (2005, January 17). Diet and Genes. *Newsweek, 145*(3), 40–42

Vacovsky, L. Finding effective treatment for alcohol dependence. *American Council on Alcoholism.* Retrieved 5/16/05, from: http://www.aca-usa.org/pharm2.htm

Williams, C. & Laird, R. (1992, Sept/Oct.) Beyond A.A. *New Age Journal,* 38.

Wilson, W. G. (1958, April 28). *Alcoholics Anonymous—Beginning and Growth.* Speech to the New York Medical Society on Alcoholism.

Wilson. W.G. (1939) *Twelve steps and twelve traditions.* New York: General Services Office, Alcoholics Anonymous

About the Author

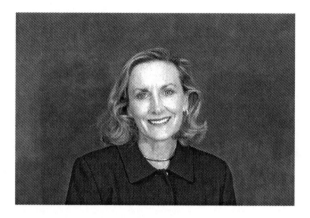

Dr. Santi Meunier has been a Psychotherapist for over 20 years helping individuals and families to recover from the devastating effects of alcoholism and other forms of addiction and abuse. She received her Doctorate in Chemical Dependency from Madison University, graduating Summa Cum Laude. Her latest book, *Dying for a Drink, The Hidden Epidemic of Alcoholism* is the result of decades of work and research in the field.

978-0-595-47396-(
0-595-47396-2

Printed in the United States
200737BV00002B/106-204/A